The Art of
LIVING AND LONGEVITY
LIVE BETTER, LONGER

Unleashing The Power Of Happiness
For a Healthier, More Fulfilling Life.

Inspired By
Peter Attia Outlive

PETER RAYMOND

Copyright © 2024 by Peter Raymond

All rights reserved. No part of this book may be reproduced or transmitted in any form or by any means, electronic or mechanical, including photocopying, recording, or by any information storage and retrieval system, without the written permission of the publisher or author, except in the case of brief quotations embodied in critical reviews and certain other noncommercial uses permitted by copyright law.

This book is published by Therapy Seminary Publishers.

Hardcover Edition: ISBN: 978-1-963674-24-8

First Edition: 2024

Disclaimer

Please note, this book is neither affiliated with nor officially endorsed by Peter Attia. It stands as a separate, independent piece, intended for informational purposes only, and not as a substitute for professional medical advice. Readers should always seek the counsel of qualified health professionals for personal health concerns.

Table of Contents

INTRODUCTION 6
WHY BOTHER READING? 8
PART 1: UNLOCKING THE SECRETS OF HAPPINESS 10
CHAPTER 1: THE HAPPINESS EQUATION 11
Defining Happiness and Its Impact on Your Life 11
Dismantling the Myths of Aging 15
Finding Your Joy: Hacking Happiness in Everyday Life 16
The Gifts of Age 18
Dave's Experience 20
CHAPTER 2: DISCOVERING YOUR JOY TRIGGERS 23
Identifying Activities and Experiences that Spark Your Inner Light 23
The Science of Joy 24
Planting the Seeds of Happiness 29
Practical Hacks from Dr. Attia 29
Your Personalized Happiness Plan 33
EXERCISE 1: Personalized Happiness Plan 35
CHAPTER 3: BEYOND RIGHT AND WRONG 44
Embracing Your Authentic Happiness Regardless of Judgment 44
Beyond the Binary 46
Jane's Experience 49
CHAPTER 4: TAMING THE INNER CRITIC 51
Silencing Negative Self-Talk and Embracing Self-Compassion 51
The Impact of Negativity on Longevity 52
Silencing the Inner Critic 53
Embracing Self-Compassion 54
The Road to Longevity and Well-being 56
EXERCISE 2: A Self-Discovery Challenge To Tame Your Inner Critic 57
PART 2: CULTIVATING HAPPINESS FOR A LONG AND FULFILLING LIFE 61

CHAPTER 5: THE HAPPINESS-LONGEVITY CONNECTION 62

How Happiness Can Add Years to Your Life and Life to Your Years 62

The Science of Happiness and Longevity 63

Happiness for a Longer, Fulfilling Life 66

Practical Ways to Cultivate Happiness 66

Felix Experience 75

CHAPTER 6: BEYOND HAPPINESS: BUILDING THE PILLARS OF WELL-BEING 78

Discovering the Relationship between Happiness, Nutrition, Exercise, and Sleep 78

Nutrition: Fueling Your Body and Mind 82

Exercise: Building a Strong Foundation 86

Sleep: The Cornerstone of Restoration and Renewal 90

CHAPTER 7: STRESS LESS, LIVE MORE 99

Practical Tools to Manage Stress and Cultivate Inner Peace 99

Understanding Stress 102

Identifying Your Stressors 102

Practical Tools for Managing Stress 104

Jane's Experience 109

CHAPTER 8: PENNYWISE, LIFEWISE 112

Making Wise Choices for Long-Term Happiness and Well-being .. 112

Ten Guiding Financial Principles 118

Longevity Goals And A Realistic Plan To Achieve Them 120

Dave's Experience 126

PART 3: LIVING A LIFE OF JOY: PUTTING IT ALL TOGETHER 129

CHAPTER 9: EMBRACING THE ZEN WITHIN 130

Integrating Mindfulness and Acceptance into Daily Life 130

Living in the "Now": The Power of Mindfulness 131

Acceptance: Embracing the Present Moment 134

EXERCISE 3: Embrace Your Inner Zen: A Fun and Practical Exercise 139

CHAPTER 10: ONE STEP AT A TIME 143
Building a Sustainable Path Towards a Happy and Fulfilling Life .143
The Power of Consistency 147
Tips to help you stay on track 148
Janes Experience 151
CHAPTER 11: THE JOURNEY CONTINUES 154
Spreading Lifetime Happiness, Embracing Continuous Growth, And Building Connections For A More Meaningful Life 154
Spreading Lifetime Happiness: The Ripple Effect of Positivity 155
CONCLUSION 160
Bonus: Q&A: Unlock Your Awesome Life 161

INTRODUCTION

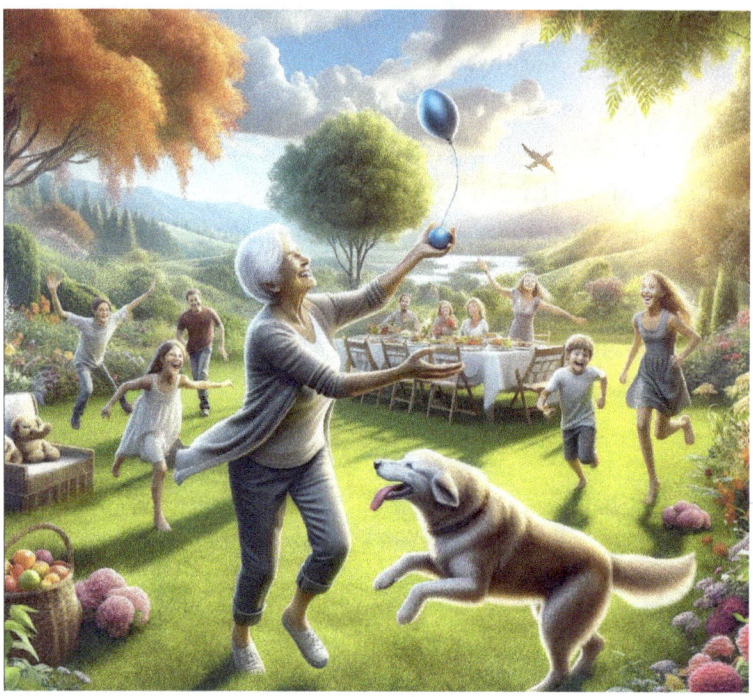

When you imagine your older self, what image comes to mind? Is it an image of you and your grandkids playing fetch with your dog in the garden? Will it be you racing your grandkids at a family get-together, just before the Thanksgiving turkey is ready to be served? Do you imagine yourself strong, healthy, with great eyesight, and unaided by a walking stick?

Or will you be hunched over, with ragged breath, aching knees, a bad bowel, regular visits to the doctor, high blood pressure, hypertension, general body weakness, largely dependent on medication, and relegated to an elderly home?

The truth is, your 80-year-old self is a blank canvas, waiting for you to paint its masterpiece. We know that the latter description is largely associated with aging, but you can design your future where your health and strength will be like that of a teenager even at 80. This isn't wishful thinking; it's the reality being embraced by a growing number of individuals rewriting the script of their aging story.

Remember Dr. Peter Attia, the renowned longevity expert. He's not just preaching – he's living proof that aging is not a disease, but a process we can influence. He's not talking about magic potions or snake oil; his approach is grounded in science, real-life examples, and actionable steps.

Guard this book jealously as the only guide you'll need to become the architect of your own longevity. I mean, wouldn't you love to still rock those stylish outfits neatly arranged in your wardrobe as a healthy granny or grandpa? It would be a wonderful time indeed...

WHY BOTHER READING?

Today, there is a notion making the rounds that the prime of life has changed. This argument states that the traditional view of aging - decline, retirement, past prime - is outdated and inaccurate. Instead, the "prime of life" has moved to our 60s and beyond. This "autumn" of life can be our richest season, full of freedom, options, wisdom, and accomplishment. By proactively planning and embracing this new prime, we can make the most of our remaining years and create a fulfilling and meaningful final chapter.

Join us as we delve into science, shattering myths and misconceptions about aging. Like the Blue Zones, communities with exceptional life expectancies, where strong social connections, active lifestyles, and plant-based diets inspire the move of longevity in action. The Framingham Heart Study, following thousands for decades, reveals how healthy habits like eating well, exercising, and maintaining a healthy weight contribute to a longer lifespan.

But it's not just about physical well-being. Happiness matters too. Studies like the Harvard Study of Adult Development show that strong social connections and positive emotions are linked to a longer life. The

Wisconsin Longitudinal Study and Nun Study confirm that experiencing joy and having a purpose in life contribute to living longer and living better.

This book is your personalized roadmap, drawing inspiration from Dr. Attia's insights. We'll equip you with practical tools to create a healthy, fulfilling future. From nutritional choices that fuel your body and exercise hacks that move joy, to mindfulness techniques that conquer stress and cultivate inner peace.

But this isn't just about adding years to your life; it's about adding life to your years. It's about embracing the adventures that await, the connections that enrich, and the experiences that make your heart sing. Imagine building a supportive community, finding your tribe, and experiencing the power of social connection.

Ready to let go of the fear of aging, living intentionally and truly happy? Turn the page, and let's jump on this journey together. Remember, your much older self is waiting - what story will you write?

PART 1: UNLOCKING THE SECRETS OF HAPPINESS

CHAPTER 1: THE HAPPINESS EQUATION
Defining Happiness and Its Impact on Your Life

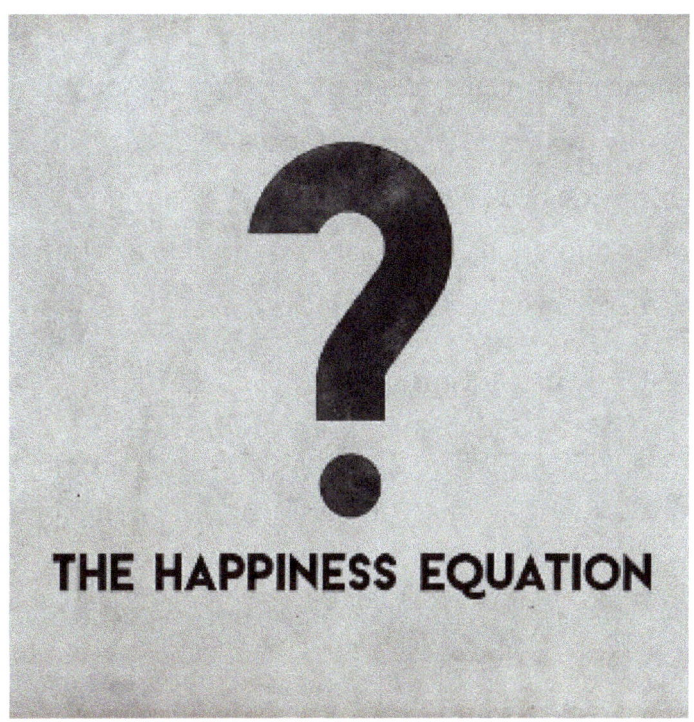

"Happiness is not a possession to be gained, but a quality of life to be cultivated." - Archbishop Desmond Tutu

Forget the Hollywood definition of happiness as a fleeting feeling of euphoria. True happiness is a deeper sense of contentment, fulfillment, and meaning in life.

It's not about constant highs, but about a general sense of peace, gratitude, and engagement with life, even when things get tough.

Studies by Dr. Sonja Lyubomirsky, a leading happiness researcher, show that happiness is about 50% influenced by genetics (your "happiness set point"), 10% by external circumstances (like wealth or relationships), and a whopping 40% by our intentional choices and actions. That means you have significant control over your own happiness!

The Happiness Equation

Here's where things get interesting. Dr. Jonathan Haidt, a renowned psychologist, suggests a "happiness equation":

$$H = S + C + V$$

- **H** stands for your overall happiness level.
- **S** represents your "happiness set point," your genetic predisposition for happiness.
- **C** represents your "life conditions," external factors like your job, relationships, and health.

- **V** represents your "voluntary activities," the choices and actions you take to cultivate happiness.

This equation highlights two key points:

1. **Happiness is multi-faceted:** It's not just about external factors or chasing fleeting emotions. It involves your genetic makeup, your life circumstances, and your own intentional efforts.

2. **You have more control than you think:** While you can't change your genes or completely control external circumstances, you have significant power over your "voluntary activities," which have a substantial impact on your happiness.

The Peter Attia Connection

As you know, Dr. Peter Attia champions a holistic approach to longevity that prioritizes both physical and mental well-being. Happiness, as defined above, fits perfectly into this framework. Studies show that happier individuals tend to live longer, healthier lives. They experience lower stress levels, stronger immune systems, and better cardiovascular health. So, cultivating happiness isn't just about feeling good, it's about living a longer, healthier life.

Cultivating Your Happiness

So, how do we put the "V" in the happiness equation? Here are some science-backed practices you can incorporate:

1. **Gratitude:** Regularly taking time to appreciate the good things in your life, big or small, has been shown to boost happiness. Try a gratitude journal or simply take a few minutes each day to reflect on what you're thankful for.
2. **Relationships:** Strong social connections are crucial for happiness. Invest in your relationships with family, friends, and loved ones. Make time for meaningful interactions, express appreciation, and offer support.
3. **Purpose:** Having a sense of purpose and meaning in life gives you direction and motivation. This could be anything from volunteering to pursuing a hobby or starting a passion project.
4. **Mindfulness:** Regularly practicing mindfulness meditation helps you become more

aware of your thoughts and emotions without judgment. This can lead to greater self-compassion, reduced stress, and increased happiness.

5. **Healthy Habits:** Taking care of your physical health through exercise, healthy eating, and good sleep also impacts your happiness. Remember, the mind and body are interconnected!

Next, let's dismantle some predominant but limiting beliefs associated with aging. Age is not a barrier to happiness; it's an opportunity to cultivate it with greater depth.

Dismantling the Myths of Aging

We're bombarded with messages equating youth with strength, success, and happiness. Our culture glorifies wrinkle-free faces and infinite energy, leaving many feeling invisible and irrelevant as they age. But before we internalize these harmful myths, let's examine them through the lens of reason and research.

The notion that happiness diminishes with age simply doesn't hold water. Studies by the National Bureau of Economic Research show that while happiness dips in midlife, it surges back in later years, surpassing even youthful levels. Why? Experience brings wisdom, self-acceptance, and deeper connections, all potent ingredients for a fulfilling life.

Another myth: your physical peak dictates your happiness. Yes, our bodies change with time, but that doesn't diminish our capacity for joy. Research by Stanford University reveals that focusing on gratitude and positive experiences outweighs the impact of physical limitations on overall well-being.

Finding Your Joy: Hacking Happiness in Everyday Life

Now that we've cleared the misconceptions, let's talk about the practical tools that can unlock your potential for happiness. Drawing upon Peter Attia's insights and evidence-based research, here are five key "happiness hacks" to cultivate as we advance in age:

1. **Relaxation and Rejuvenation:** Ditch the chronic stress and prioritize self-care. Meditation, mindfulness exercises, and spending time in nature are powerful tools for de-stressing and recharging your inner batteries.
2. **Reflection and Recollection:** Savor the richness of your journey. Spend time reminiscing about cherished memories,

journaling your experiences, and appreciating the lessons learned. This fosters a sense of purpose and gratitude for the life you've built.

3. **Relationships and Reconciliation:** Nurture the connections that matter most. Invest time in deepening relationships with loved ones, mend past hurts, and build new bonds. Strong social connections are the bedrock of happiness in later life.

4. **Repentance and Restitution:** Make peace with your past. Acknowledge mistakes, forgive yourself and others, and strive to make amends where possible. This frees you from burdens and allows you to live with greater authenticity and inner peace.

5. **Reinvention and Re-creation:** Embrace the power of reinvention. Explore new passions, learn new skills, and challenge yourself to step outside your comfort zone. This keeps you engaged, motivated, and excited about the future.

Remember, these "hacks" are not one-time fixes, but ongoing practices that become habits, weaving themselves into the tapestry of your daily life.

The Gifts of Age

Think aging is simply about deterioration? Think again! As we advance in age, it comes with its own unique set of advantages:

1. **Freedom and Flexibility:** You're likely no longer constrained by the demands of career and childcare, freeing you to pursue passions and explore new possibilities.
2. **Time and Choice:** With more control over your time, you can prioritize activities that bring you joy and meaning, creating a life less rushed and more intentional.
3. **Depth and Perspective:** Years of experience grant you valuable wisdom and the ability to see things with a broader lens. This fosters resilience, compassion, and a deeper understanding of yourself and the world.
4. **Gratitude and Contentment:** With a fuller life lived, you gain a profound appreciation for what you have, shifting your focus from chasing more to cherishing what truly matters.
5. **Relationships and Legacy:** The bonds you've nurtured over time deepen and become sources of immense strength and joy. You have the

opportunity to leave a lasting legacy through your wisdom, love, and the connections you've built.

The good news aging brings is that happiness isn't reserved for the chosen few. It is attainable by anyone willing to consciously invest time and effort.

Remember, you are not defined by your age but by the richness of your experiences and the potential you hold within. It's never too late to rewrite the story of your life and claim your well-deserved happiness.

Forget the tired narrative of "life is what happens." This book is for those who believe the past is just the prologue, not the whole story.

Are you ready to unlock a future where you don't just survive, you thrive?

This isn't another book filled with limitations. It's your roadmap to turning a long life into your greatest adventure, not a burden.

Packed with actionable insights, it's an invitation to own your journey, explore your options, and shape your future, today.

Ready to ditch the "curse" and embrace the "gift"?

Then join us on this exciting exploration and let's rewrite your story together.

Dave's Experience

The first wrinkle I saw wasn't on my face, it was on my driver's license. 40. Forty? In my mind, I was still that 25-year-old graduate fresh from the university (been stuck in this narrative for so many years), fueled by ambition. Now, here I was, staring at the stark evidence time awarded me. I had a panic attack, I had never really experienced true happiness and my life is rolling by and I am just a spectator. Where did my youth go?

I became terrified of birthdays. Each year felt like a countdown, not to some grand celebration, but to the inevitable decline. The wrinkles multiplied, creaking knees, and the dreaded "senior discount" loomed like vultures circling a carcass. It wasn't until I stumbled upon the research of Peter Attia, a longevity doctor with a refreshingly irreverent approach to aging, that I dared to reframe my perspective.

See, Attia doesn't sugarcoat the biological realities of aging, but he also doesn't subscribe to the cultural narrative of inevitable misery. His message resonated:

happiness isn't a finite resource that dwindles with each passing year; it's a skill, and like any skill, it can be honed with practice.

Now, before you roll your eyes and mutter "easier said than done," let me tell you about Uncle Frank. Frank, God bless his soul, was the epitome of a grumpy old man. He complained about everything, from the price of milk to the color of the sky. He also hated the idea of marking his birthdays, he said it only reminded him of how close he was to his grave.

Then, one day, Frank turned 75. Instead of the usual grumbling, he told me he was taking up tango lessons. Tango? The man who couldn't walk a block without complaining? It seemed ridiculous, yet there he was, shuffling awkwardly across the dance floor, a goofy grin plastered on his face.

Turns out, tango wasn't just about the steps; it was about connection, laughter, and the sheer joy of trying something new. Frank, the man who seemed perpetually on the verge of a major meltdown, was radiating happiness. It was a revelation.

His story gave me hope. If Frank, the walking embodiment of negativity, could find joy as he grew older, then surely I could too. He told me it wasn't about defying the aging process; it was about embracing it, flaws and all.

I know aging isn't all sunshine and rainbows. There will be days my joints will ache, and the mirror shows me a stranger. But I also know that with each year I get to understand myself better, find wisdom in my experiences, and have the freedom to prioritize what truly matters.

This journey isn't about chasing some elusive fountain of youth; it's about finding the humor in the wrinkles and the joy in simply being alive. And that, my friends, is a quest worth celebrating, regardless of the number on the cake.

Now, if you'll excuse me, I have a tango lesson to catch. Just don't expect any fancy footwork – I'm more of a two-left-feet kinda gal. But hey, at least I'm having fun. And that, in the end, is all that matters.

CHAPTER 2: DISCOVERING YOUR JOY TRIGGERS
Identifying Activities and Experiences that Spark Your Inner Light

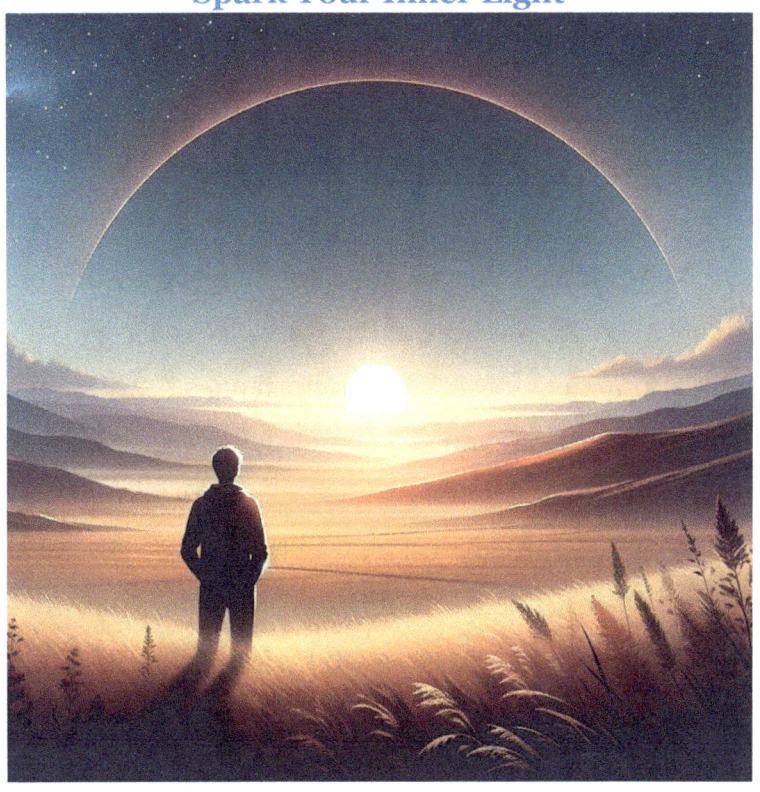

"Joy is not in things, it is in us." - John Ruskin

Life's journey is filled with highs and lows, yet cultivating joy and inner light within ourselves strengthens our resilience and fosters longevity. Dr.

Peter Attia emphasizes the importance of self-discovery and identifying personal "joy triggers" – activities and experiences that ignite happiness and fulfillment. These triggers fuel our intrinsic well-being, influencing not only our mood but also potentially impacting our physical health and longevity.

The Science of Joy

Science tells us that joy has profound effects on our brains and bodies. When we engage in activities that spark joy, dopamine and serotonin, neurotransmitters associated with pleasure and reward, are released. This activation can lower stress hormones, strengthen immune function, and even potentially reduce the risk of chronic diseases. Dr. Attia, referring to research by Dr. Robert Waldinger, director of the Harvard Study of Adult Development, highlights the link between positive emotions and longevity: "Individuals who find their joy triggers and regularly experience joy tend to live longer and healthier lives."

Identifying Your Joy Triggers

Discovering your unique joy triggers requires exploration and experimentation. Here are some steps to guide you:

1. **Mindfulness**: Pay attention to your internal compass. Notice activities, moments, and environments that naturally uplift your mood and leave you feeling energized and satisfied.

2. **Reflection**: Consider past experiences. Recall memories when you felt truly joyful and analyze what contributed to that feeling. Was it spending time in nature, pursuing a creative hobby, connecting with loved ones, or achieving a personal goal?

Take some quiet time to ask yourself these questions:

- *What did I enjoy doing as a kid, before the pressures of adulthood took over?*

- *What activities make me lose myself in the moment, forgetting about time and worries?*

- *What accomplishments bring me a deep sense of satisfaction?*

- *What kind of impact do I want to have on the world?*

- *What values are most important to me, and how can I live them out more fully?*

3. **Variety**: Don't limit yourself! Try new things, even if they seem outside your comfort zone. You might discover unexpected sources of joy.

4. **Intentionality**: Schedule time for activities you suspect might bring you joy. This could be anything from reading a book in a park to trying a new recipe to taking a dance class.

5. **Observation**: Notice how you feel during and after each activity. Did it energize you? Did it leave you feeling calm and content? Did it spark creativity or motivation?

6. **Refine**: Based on your observations, refine your understanding of your joy triggers. Identify patterns and common threads that connect these activities.

Examples of Joy Triggers

- **Movement and Connection:** Engaging in physical activities like sports, dancing, or hiking can promote joy and release endorphins. Equally important, connecting with loved ones through shared experiences fosters social connection and reduces stress.

- **Creativity and Learning:** Immersing ourselves in creative pursuits like art, music, or writing can provide self-expression and a sense of accomplishment. Likewise, continuous learning through reading, documentaries, or courses stimulates the mind and sparks curiosity.

- **Nature and Giving Back:** Spending time in nature has been shown to reduce stress, enhance mood, and promote mindfulness. Engaging in activities that benefit others, like volunteering or helping a neighbor, can cultivate happiness and purpose.

Remember, your joy triggers are unique to you. What brings joy to one person might not do the same for another. What matters most is that you actively seek out and engage in activities that resonate with your values and interests.

Making joy a priority isn't a self-indulgent luxury; it's an investment in your well-being and longevity. By identifying and incorporating your joy triggers into your life, you cultivate a richer, more fulfilling experience and pave the way for a healthier, happier future.

Planting the Seeds of Happiness
Practical Hacks from Dr. Attia

Once you have a clearer understanding of your "joy soil," it's time to plant the seeds that will blossom into a fulfilling life. Dr. Attia, drawing on his expertise and the wisdom of countless individuals, offers some practical "happiness hacks":

- **Gratitude is your fertilizer:** Take time each day to appreciate the good things in your life, big and small. A grateful heart finds joy in the present moment, regardless of circumstances.

- **Relationships are your sunshine:** Nurture your connections with loved ones, build new friendships, and engage in activities that strengthen your bonds. Strong relationships are a powerful source of happiness and support.

- **Move your body, move your mood:** Regular physical activity is a well-known mood booster. Find activities you enjoy, whether it's dancing, swimming, walking, or simply stretching.

- **Challenge your mind, challenge your joy:** Keep your brain sharp and engaged by learning new skills, taking up a hobby, or reading books that challenge and inspire you.

- **Give back and watch your joy grow:** Volunteering your time and talents to others not only benefits them but also creates a sense of purpose and connection, boosting your own happiness.

- **Sleep is your watering can:** Chronic sleep deprivation wreaks havoc on your mood and well-being. Aim for 7-8 hours of quality sleep each night.

- **Manage stress, nurture your happiness:** Stress is a happiness killer. Practice relaxation techniques like meditation, deep breathing, or spending time in nature.

- **Celebrate the small wins:** Don't wait for grand achievements to celebrate. Acknowledge and appreciate your progress, no matter how small.

Remember, this is not a rigid rulebook. Experiment, mix, and match, and find what works best for you. The key is to be intentional about creating a life that nourishes your unique joy.

Growing Beyond the Weeds: Overcoming Challenges

Let's be honest, life throws curveballs. There will be times when negativity creeps in, threatening to choke out your happiness garden. But don't despair! Dr. Attia emphasizes the importance of resilience and finding growth even in challenges. Here are some tips for navigating the weeds:

1. **Acknowledge your emotions:** Don't bottle up your feelings. Talk to someone you trust, write them down, or express them through creative outlets.

2. **Seek support:** Don't be afraid to ask for help from friends, family, or professionals when you need it.

3. **Rethink your negative thoughts**: Dr. Attia emphasizes this as a powerful tool for cultivating happiness. Here are some strategies:

   - **Challenge those inner critics:** When negative thoughts pop up, challenge them with evidence. Are they truly accurate? Are they helping you? Talk back to them with a compassionate voice and remind yourself of your strengths and accomplishments.

- **Flip the script:** Try reframing negative situations into opportunities for growth. For example, instead of viewing a setback as a failure, see it as a chance to learn and improve.

- **Focus on what you can control:** Dwelling on things outside your control only adds to stress. Focus your energy on things you can influence, like your thoughts, actions, and reactions.

- **Practice gratitude, even in tough times:** Finding something to be grateful for, even amidst challenges, can shift your perspective and boost your mood.

Remember, there will be sunny days and rainy days, but by understanding your "joy blueprint," planting the seeds of positive habits, and overcoming challenges with resilience, you can design a life that blooms with happiness and fulfillment.

Your Personalized Happiness Plan

Now it's your turn! Take what you've learned and create your own personalized happiness plan. Here are some steps to get you started:

1. **Reflect on your current state:** How happy are you on a scale of 1-10? What are the biggest contributors to your happiness? What areas could use some improvement?

2. **Review your "joy blueprint":** What activities truly light you up? What values do you want to live by?

3. **Choose 3-5 "happiness hacks" to implement:** Pick a few strategies from Dr. Attia's suggestions or come up with your own.

4. **Set SMART goals:** Make your goals Specific, Measurable, Achievable, Relevant, and Time-bound. For example, instead of saying "I want to be happier," aim for "I will spend 15 minutes each day doing a mindful activity like meditation."

5. **Take action!:** Start implementing your plan and track your progress. Celebrate your successes along the way!

Remember, this is your journey, and there's no one-size-fits-all approach. Be patient, experiment, and have fun! As Dr. Attia reminds us, "Longevity is not just about living longer, it's about living better." And living better starts with designing a life that sparks your unique joy.

EXERCISE 1: Personalized Happiness Plan

Are you ready to nurture your inner light and design a life that sparks genuine happiness? This exercise will guide you through Dr. Attia's insights, helping you identify your unique "joy triggers" and build a personalized plan for lasting fulfillment.

Step 1: Reflect & Recharge (10 minutes)

- **Happiness Meter:** Rate your current happiness on a scale of 1-10.

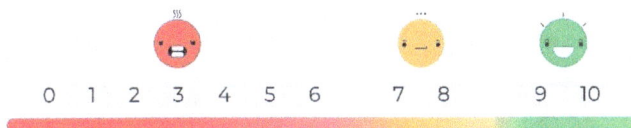

- What factors contribute most to your joy?

_____
_____
_____
_____
_____
_____
_____

- Are there areas you'd like to improve?

_____

_____

_____

_____

_____

_____

_____

- **Memory Lane:** Close your eyes and recall a time when you felt truly joyful. What elements contributed to that feeling? Was it spending time with loved ones, achieving a goal, or simply immersing yourself in a cherished activity?

_____

_____

_____

_____

_____

_____

Step 2: Discover Your Joy Blueprint (15 minutes)

- **Mindful Moments:** Throughout the day, pay attention to activities that naturally uplift your mood. What sparks a sense of energy, satisfaction, or fulfillment? Write down these "joy triggers" as you discover them.

_____
_____
_____
_____
_____
_____
_____
_____
_____
_____
_____
_____

- **Question to reflect on:**
    - What are some of the things you enjoyed doing as a child before adult pressures took over?

_____
_____

_____
_____
_____
_____
_____

- What activities make you lose track of time and forget about worries?

_____
_____
_____
_____
_____

- What accomplishments bring you deep satisfaction?

_____
_____
_____
_____
_____

- What kind of impact do you want to have on the world?

  _____
  _____
  _____
  _____
  _____

- What values are most important to you, and how can you live them out more fully?

  _____
  _____
  _____
  _____
  _____

Step 3: Design Your Happiness Garden (20 minutes)

- **Choose Your Seeds:** Pick 3-5 "happiness hacks" from Dr. Attia's suggestions or create your own based on your joy triggers.

Consider:

- **Gratitude:** What simple things can you appreciate daily?

- **Relationships:** How can you strengthen existing connections and build new ones?

- **Movement:** What physical activities bring you joy and energize you?

- **Challenges:** How can you learn something new or take on a stimulating challenge?

  _____
  _____
  _____
  _____
  _____

- **Giving Back:** How can you volunteer your time or talents to benefit others?

  _____
  _____
  _____
  _____
  _____

- **Sleep:** Are you prioritizing quality sleep for optimal well-being?

  _____
  _____
  _____
  _____
  _____

- **Stress Management:** What relaxation techniques can you incorporate into your life?

- **Celebrate Wins:** How will you acknowledge and appreciate your progress, big or small?

Step 4: Plant & Grow (Unending)

- **SMART Goals:** Make your happiness hacks specific, measurable, achievable, relevant, and time-bound. For example, instead of "be more social," aim for "join a local book club next month."

- **Take Action!:** Start implementing your personalized plan and track your progress. Use a journal, or app, or simply check in with yourself regularly.

- **Celebrate & Adapt:** Acknowledge your successes, no matter how small. Be patient, experiment, and adjust your plan as needed. Remember, joy is a journey, not a destination!

Share your journey! Connect with others on their happiness paths and inspire each other to cultivate joy-filled lives.

Remember, this is YOUR unique plan. Embrace the process, have fun, and let your inner light shine!

CHAPTER 3: BEYOND RIGHT AND WRONG
Embracing Your Authentic Happiness Regardless of Judgment

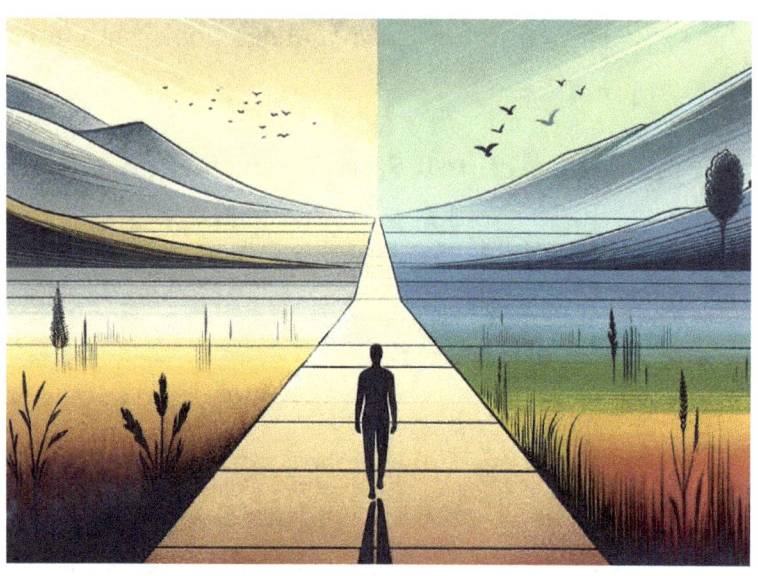

"One who looks around him is intelligent, one who looks within him is wise."
-Matshona Dhliwayo

Remember the story of the two arrows? When misfortune strikes, the first arrow is the event itself, unavoidable and beyond our control. But the second arrow, the sting of suffering, is optional. It's our thoughts and judgments about the event that creates the pain, not the event itself. This chapter welcomes you to leave the judgment train behind and embark on a journey toward authentic happiness, free from the constraints of right and wrong.

The Deception of Dualism

We're wired to categorize, judge, and label. We see the world through a binary lens of right and wrong, good and bad, success and failure. This can help make quick decisions, but it also creates a rigid framework that limits our happiness and well-being. It's important to remember that these labels are often subjective and culturally influenced, not absolute truths.

The Perception Trap

Think back to your favorite coffee shop. One person might be having an existential crisis, while another enjoys their latte in blissful peace. Both are experiencing the same physical environment, yet their internal worlds are vastly different. This illustrates how our perception, shaped by thoughts and judgments, creates our reality. The event itself is neutral; it's our interpretation that determines our emotional response.

The Thought Experiment

Imagine you hate your job. It fills you with stress and anxiety. Now, ask yourself: who would you be without that thought? Take a moment to truly explore this question. Without the judgment of "hating" your job, you might find feelings of freedom, peace, and lightness emerge. This simple exercise demonstrates the power our thoughts have over our emotions and experiences.

Beyond the Binary

Judgment isn't inherently bad. It can help us navigate complex situations and make ethical choices. However, when we cling to rigid judgments, we miss the complexities of life. Instead of labeling things as "good" or "bad," try to see them on a spectrum. This allows for greater understanding and compassion, both for ourselves and others.

The Power of Reframing

Instead of dwelling on the negative aspects of a situation, try reframing it in a more positive light. Look for the silver linings, the opportunities for growth, and the lessons learned. This shift in perspective can significantly impact your emotional state and overall well-being.

Embrace Imperfection

The pursuit of perfection is a recipe for disappointment. We all make mistakes, experience setbacks, and have flaws. Instead of judging yourself harshly, learn to accept and embrace your imperfections. This self-compassion is essential for authentic happiness and inner peace.

Find Your Authentic Self

Let go of societal expectations and external pressures. What truly matters to you? What brings you joy and fulfillment? Connect with your inner voice and values, and allow them to guide your choices. This authenticity is the foundation of true happiness.

Live in the Present Moment

Our minds often dwell on the past or worry about the future, missing the beauty and richness of the present moment. Mindfulness practices like meditation and deep breathing can help you anchor yourself in the present and appreciate what life offers right now.

Happiness is not a fixed state, but an ongoing journey. There will be ups and downs, challenges and triumphs. The key is to embrace the journey, learn from experiences, and keep moving forward with a growth mindset.

Remember:

- You are not your thoughts.
- Judgments are subjective perceptions, not absolute truths.
- You have the power to reframe your thinking and choose your emotional response.
- Authentic happiness comes from accepting yourself, embracing imperfections, and living in the present moment.

Imagine life beyond just "right" and "wrong." This isn't about ignoring morals, but seeing them as stepping stones, not walls. Our struggles don't define us, it's how we interpret them that creates suffering. Think of your mind as a garden. You can grow negativity or joy, the choice is yours.

Instead of silencing your thoughts, understand their power and choose wisely. See challenges as opportunities, and setbacks as lessons. Every thought holds the potential to shift your world. Choose thoughts that fuel happiness, passion, and your true self.

This journey isn't about blame, but about unlocking the wisdom within. You deserve happiness, and the key lies not in external circumstances, but in the garden you cultivate within your mind. So, breathe deeply, choose wisely, and watch your life blossom.

Jane's Experience

My name is Jane Richmond, at the age of 42 I became a single mom and CEO of a drowning company, and I was deeply stressed. My mind, a relentless judge, labeled everything "wrong" – my job, lack of time, failed relationship, etc. I felt trapped in a double world, constantly striving for an impossible perfection.

Then, a mindfulness course opened a door. It wasn't about silencing thoughts but understanding their power. It taught me to see challenges as opportunities, and setbacks as lessons. For the first time, I questioned the "wrongness" of my situation. Was it truly bad, or just my interpretation?

The shift was quiet, yet profound. I started noticing the good amidst the chaos – the supportive colleagues, the resilience of my child, the quiet moments of joy. My judgmental lens softened, replaced by curiosity and compassion. I even began to see the "wrong" choices as stepping stones, leading me to unexpected growth.

It wasn't easy. The judging voice still whispered, but now, I have the tools to silence it. I now choose thoughts that fuel happiness, not self-criticism. I see my "imperfections" as an opportunity the universe is presenting to me to be better, and not as flaws. And most importantly, I learned to live in the present moment, savoring the small victories and finding peace amidst the chaos.

My journey isn't about ignoring right and wrong, but about embracing the spectrum in between. It's about understanding that happiness doesn't lie in external circumstances, but in the garden I cultivate within my mind.

So, if you're struggling with judgment, remember my story. Choose wisely, nurture your inner garden, and watch your life blossom beyond the confines of right and wrong. You deserve happiness, and it's waiting to be discovered within.

CHAPTER 4: TAMING THE INNER CRITIC
Silencing Negative Self-Talk and Embracing Self-Compassion

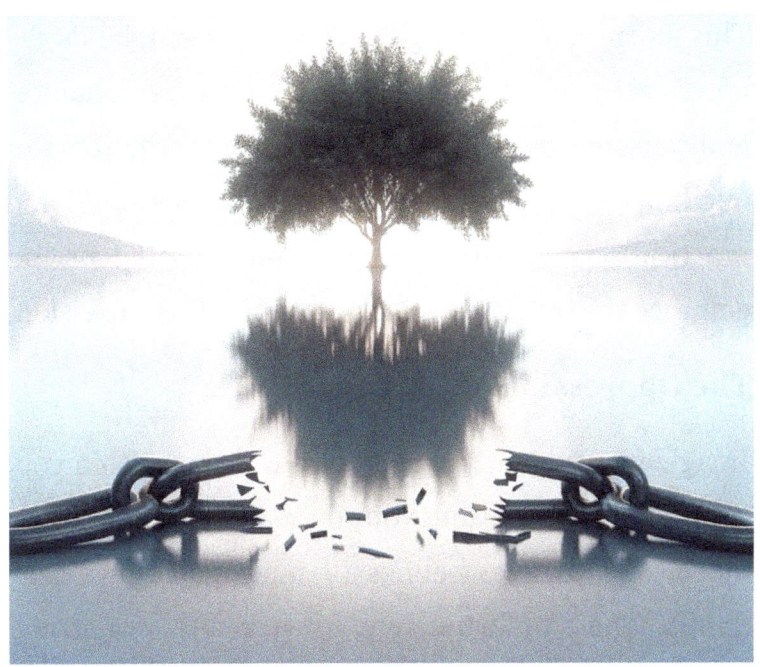

"Your health and happiness are directly impacted by your inner dialogue."
-Peter Attia, M.D.

As Peter Attia aptly states, "The mind is a powerful tool. But like any tool, it can be used for good or for harm." Perhaps nowhere is this truer than in the circle of our inner dialogue. The constant chatter of self-criticism, doubt, and negativity can be a relentless source of suffering, chipping away at our confidence and well-being. But what if we could learn to silence this inner critic and cultivate self-compassion instead?

This journey, as challenging as it may seem, holds the potential to unlock a deeper sense of peace, acceptance, and personal growth. Here, we'll explore the roots of our inner critic, the impact of negative self-talk, and practical strategies to tame this internal saboteur and embrace the transformative power of self-compassion.

The Oppression of the Inner Critic

Imagine a constant, critical voice residing within you, relentlessly pointing out your flaws, judging your every move, and fueling feelings of inadequacy and self-doubt. This, unfortunately, is a reality for many individuals. The inner critic, a collection of negative thoughts and beliefs formed through past experiences and societal conditioning, acts as a self-sabotaging force. It whispers negativity, amplifies our shortcomings, and fuels anxieties and insecurities.

The Impact of Negativity on Longevity
Chronic negativity isn't just emotionally draining; it can also have detrimental effects on our physical

health. Studies have linked excessive self-criticism to increased stress hormones, weakened immune systems, and a higher risk of chronic diseases like heart disease and depression. Additionally, the stress response triggered by a critical inner voice can lead to unhealthy behaviors like overeating, alcohol abuse, and sleep disturbances, further jeopardizing our well-being and longevity.

Silencing the Inner Critic

So, how do we silence this nagging voice and reclaim our inner peace? The good news is, we have more power than we realize. Here are some potent strategies to tame your inner critic:

1. **Awareness is Key:** The first step is to become aware of your inner critic's presence. Pay attention to your self-talk. When do you hear this critical voice? What triggers it? Identifying the patterns is crucial for addressing them effectively.
2. **Challenge Its Authority:** Don't blindly accept your inner critic's pronouncements. Ask yourself: "Is this thought true? Is it helpful? Would I speak to a friend this way?" Challenge its negativity with logic and reason.

3. **Reframe Your Thinking:** Instead of dwelling on what's wrong, reframe your thoughts to focus on your strengths and accomplishments. Celebrate your victories, big and small. Gratitude practice can be a powerful tool for shifting your perspective towards appreciation.

4. **Practice Self-Compassion:** Treat yourself with the same kindness and understanding you would offer a dear friend. Acknowledge your imperfections and shortcomings without judgment. Remember, everyone makes mistakes; it's part of being human.

5. **Seek Support:** Talking to a trusted friend, therapist, or counselor can provide valuable support and guidance in managing your inner critic. Sharing your struggles and receiving objective feedback can empower you to develop healthier coping mechanisms.

Embracing Self-Compassion

Taming the inner critic is about more than just silencing negative thoughts; it's about cultivating self-compassion. Self-compassion is the practice of treating yourself with the same kindness, understanding, and acceptance you would offer to someone you care about.

It fosters emotional resilience, promotes self-forgiveness, and allows you to navigate life's challenges with greater ease.

Here are some practices to cultivate self-compassion:

1. **Mindfulness:** Mindfulness meditation helps you become aware of your thoughts and feelings without judgment. Through practice, you can learn to observe your inner critic with detachment and choose how to respond instead of being automatically controlled by it.

2. **Loving-Kindness Meditation:** This practice involves sending yourself and others well wishes like "May I be happy, may I be healthy, may I be safe." It cultivates a sense of warmth and kindness towards yourself, fostering self-acceptance and reducing self-criticism.

3. **Practice Gratitude:** Focusing on the good things in your life, big and small, shifts your perspective towards appreciation and fosters a sense of contentment. Keeping a gratitude journal or expressing gratitude to others can be powerful tools for self-compassion.

The Road to Longevity and Well-being

Taming the inner critic and embracing self-compassion are not quick fixes; they require commitment and consistent practice. However, the rewards are enormous. By silencing the negativity and nurturing self-acceptance, you embark on a journey towards greater emotional well-being, resilience, and ultimately, a more fulfilling and longer life. Remember, you are not alone in this journey. By understanding your inner critic, using the tools provided, and seeking support when needed, you can cultivate the self-compassion that paves the way for a more peaceful, joyful, and ultimately, longer life.

EXERCISE 2: A Self-Discovery Challenge To Tame Your Inner Critic

Instructions:

Grab a pen, paper, and your favorite beverage (tea, coffee, or even a glass of water!) and get ready to embark on a journey of self-discovery!

As you read through the following questions, reflect on your inner critic and how it impacts your thoughts, feelings, and behaviors. Be honest with yourself, but also remember to be kind. This is a chance to learn and grow, not to judge.

Questions:

1. **Identify your inner critic.** What does it sound like? What are its favorite things to say to you? When do you hear it most often?

_____
_____
_____
_____
_____
_____

2. **Think about the impact of your inner critic.** How does it make you feel? How does it affect your behavior?

_____
_____
_____
_____
_____
_____

3. **Choose one of the strategies mentioned in the chapter to challenge your inner critic.** How can you put this strategy into practice in your own life?

_____
_____
_____
_____
_____

4. **Imagine a situation where you typically hear your inner critic.** How would you respond to this situation differently if you were practicing self-compassion?

_____
_____
_____
_____
_____
_____
_____
_____
_____
_____

5. **Reflect on your progress.** What are some challenges you have faced in taming your inner critic? What successes have you had?

_____
_____

6. **Create a visual representation of your inner critic.** What does it look like? What does it symbolize?

7. **Write a letter to your inner critic.** Express your understanding and desire to change your relationship with it.

_____

_____

_____

Share your experiences and insights with others who are on the same journey. Don't be afraid to ask for help. There are many resources available to support you on your journey to self-compassion.

Remember, taming your inner critic is a journey, not a destination. Be patient with yourself, celebrate your successes, and don't give up!

PART 2: CULTIVATING HAPPINESS FOR A LONG AND FULFILLING LIFE

CHAPTER 5: THE HAPPINESS-LONGEVITY CONNECTION
How Happiness Can Add Years to Your Life and Life to Your Years

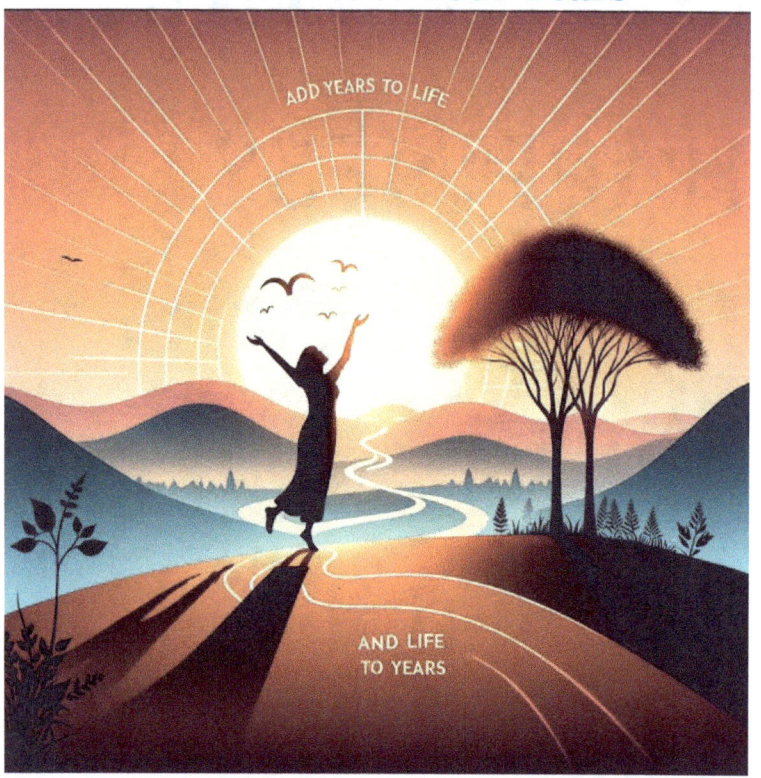

"Happiness is not a possession, it is a quality of life."
- Aristotle

This quote by the ancient Greek philosopher resonates deeply with the emerging science of happiness and its connection to longevity. While we often think of happiness as a fleeting feeling, research suggests it's much more: a potent force shaping our physical and mental well-being, potentially even influencing how long we live. Let's see how happiness connects with longevity and how we can tap into this gift to add years to your life and life to your years.

The Science of Happiness and Longevity

Understanding the science behind happiness is key to finding practical ways to increase it. Here's what science tells us:

- **Happier People Live Longer**: Longitudinal studies like the landmark Nun Study revealed a strong correlation between happiness and longevity. Nuns who reported higher levels of positive emotions lived significantly longer than those with less cheerful dispositions.

- **Happiness Protects Against Disease:** Happy individuals have more robust immune systems, suggesting they might be better equipped to fight off illness. They also tend to exhibit healthier behaviors, influencing reduced risks of chronic conditions.

- **Genetics and Temperament**: While genetics play a role, a significant portion of your happiness is within your control.

- **The Hedonic Treadmill**: We tend to adapt quickly to positive life circumstances, meaning that seeking only external pleasures won't lead to lasting happiness.

- **Happiness is a Skill**: Happiness can be learned and cultivated through deliberate practice and intentional activities.

- **Happiness Buffers Stress**: Positive emotions can counteract the negative effects of stress, a major risk factor for various health problems.

Dr. Attia, a physician and podcast host known for his deep dives into longevity research, frequently emphasizes the mind-body connection. He highlights studies demonstrating how happiness can impact various aspects of health, including:

- **Reduced stress:** Happiness is linked to lower levels of cortisol, a stress hormone known to negatively affect immune function, blood pressure, and cardiovascular health.

- **Inflammation:** Positive emotions can dampen inflammation, a chronic condition associated with numerous age-related diseases.

- **Healthy behaviors:** Happy individuals are more likely to engage in healthy behaviors like regular exercise, a balanced diet, and quality sleep, all crucial for longevity.

- **Immune system function:** Happiness has been shown to boost immune response, helping the body fight off infections and diseases.

Beyond the individual studies, a growing body of research paints a clear picture: individuals who experience higher levels of happiness tend to live longer and healthier lives. A 2023 meta-analysis published in the journal "Nature Aging" found that happier people had a 10% lower risk of early death compared to their less happy counterparts. Studies by Dr. Edward Diener, a leading happiness researcher, have revealed similar trends, demonstrating a link between happiness and longevity across various demographics.

But how does this work? Dr. Attia often suggests multiple mechanisms at play. Happiness might directly influence biological processes like inflammation and stress response. It could also indirectly promote longevity by encouraging healthy lifestyle choices and fostering stronger social connections, both crucial for well-being and longevity.

Happiness for a Longer, Fulfilling Life

While the science is compelling, it's natural to wonder how to translate this knowledge into practical action. Fortunately, Dr. Attia and other longevity experts offer valuable insights:

Key components of happiness:

- **Hedonic Well-being**: This refers to the positive, pleasurable experiences and emotions we feel in the moment.

- **Eudaimonic Well-being**: This deeper type of happiness stems from living a meaningful and purposeful life aligned with your values.

- **Social Well-Being**: Fostering strong connections and a sense of belonging is crucial.

Practical Ways to Cultivate Happiness

Now let's dive into specific, science-backed strategies to boost happiness and well-being:

1. **Social Connection**

   - The Science: Strong social bonds are one of the most significant predictors of happiness and longevity. They improve resilience and provide support.

   - Putting it into Practice:

     - Cultivate Relationships: Prioritize quality time with loved ones, share experiences, and offer support.

     - Join a Club or Group: Pursue interests with like-minded people, build new connections, and a sense of community.

     - Volunteer: Help others in need; this boosts both their happiness and yours.

2. **Acts of Kindness**

   - The Science: Kindness activates reward centers in the brain, fosters empathy, and strengthens social bonds.

   - Putting it into Practice:

- Small Gestures: Practice random acts of kindness like paying for someone's coffee or offering a compliment.
- Pay It Forward: Start a chain reaction of kindness by helping someone and asking them to do the same for others.
- Volunteer Your Time: Dedicate time to a cause you care about.

3. Gratitude

- The Science: Gratitude increases activity in brain regions associated with reward and positive emotions. It strengthens optimism and resilience.
- Putting it into Practice:
  - Keep a Gratitude Journal: Write down three things you're grateful for each day.
  - Thank-You Notes: Express gratitude to someone who's made a positive difference in your life.

- Savor the Good: Take a few minutes to consciously appreciate positive experiences as they happen.

4. **Positive Thinking**

- The Science: Optimism is linked to better physical and mental health, and greater resilience in the face of challenges.

- Putting it into Practice:

    - Challenge Negative Thoughts: Examine your automatic thoughts and reframe them into more realistic and positive interpretations.

    - Best Possible Self: Practice visualizing and writing about your best possible future self.

    - Positive Reappraisal: Look for the silver lining in difficult situations, focusing on what you can learn and how you can grow.

5. **Mindfulness and Meditation**

- The Science: Mindfulness reduces stress, increases focus, and cultivates self-awareness.

Meditation can alter brain structure in areas associated with well-being.

- Putting it into Practice:
  - Mindfulness Exercises: Practice focusing on your breath, body sensations, or present-moment experiences without judgment.
  - Meditation Apps: Utilize guided meditations like those available in Headspace or Calm.
  - Walking Meditation: Consciously focus on your surroundings and sensations as you walk.

6. Flow States

  - The Science: Flow is a state of complete absorption in an activity, leading to a sense of enjoyment, focus, and loss of self-consciousness.

7. Fostering Strong Relationships

  - Invest in Quality Time: Put effort into connecting with loved ones. Prioritize

meaningful conversations and enjoyable activities together.
- Nurture Supportive Friendships: Surround yourself with positive, caring people. True friends provide support, laughter, and a sense of belonging.
- Practice Forgiveness: Letting go of grudges and resentments frees you from emotional burdens and fosters healthier relationships.
- Resolve Conflicts Constructively: Work on communication and problem-solving skills for healthier conflict resolution in your relationships.

8. Prioritizing Sleep

- Aim for 7-8 Hours: Consistent, quality sleep is vital for physical and emotional well-being. Having a set sleep and wake time is beneficial.
- Create a Relaxing Bedtime Routine: Engage in calming activities before bed, such as taking a warm bath, reading, or listening to soothing music.

- Make Your Bedroom Sleep-Conducive: Ensure your room is dark, quiet, and cool for optimal sleep conditions.

9. Healthy Nourishment

- Whole Foods Diet: Focus on fruits, vegetables, whole grains, and lean proteins. Limit processed foods, sugary drinks, and unhealthy fats.

- Mindful Eating: Pay attention to your food, savoring textures and flavors without distractions. This improves both digestion and appreciation for meals.

- Stay Hydrated: Proper hydration is crucial for physical health and even influences cognitive functioning.

10. Challenging Yourself

- Embrace Lifelong Learning: Cultivate a sense of curiosity by taking classes, reading, or learning new skills. This keeps your mind active and engaged.

- Set Attainable Goals: Working towards goals provides direction and a sense of accomplishment, both of which boost happiness. Break large goals into smaller, achievable steps to stay motivated.

- Step Outside Your Comfort Zone: Take on manageable challenges in a safe environment. Stepping outside your usual routine builds confidence and resilience.

11. Managing Stress

- Stress-Reduction Techniques: Regular practices like yoga, deep breathing, or progressive muscle relaxation can help manage stress.

- Seek Professional Help if Needed: If you're struggling with chronic stress or anxiety, reach out to a therapist or counselor who can provide guidance and coping mechanisms.

- Find Healthy Outlets: Express yourself through creative activities or exercise to release stress and boost your mood.

12. Putting it into Practice:

- Skill-Challenge Balance: Engage in activities that are slightly challenging but match your skill level.

- Clear Goals and Feedback: Have defined objectives and ways to measure progress in your chosen activity.

- Minimize Distractions: Create an environment that facilitates concentration and allows you to focus on the task at hand.

In conclusion, what works for one person may not work for another. Find practices that resonate with you and tailor them to your lifestyle. Focus on creating sustainable habits rather than drastic changes. Small, consistent actions contribute to lasting happiness.

Cultivating happiness takes ongoing effort and dedication. Don't get discouraged by setbacks; instead, view them as learning opportunities.

While these practices strongly increase the likelihood of greater happiness and fulfillment, there is no single strategy that guarantees absolute bliss for everyone.

While living longer is a worthy goal, Dr. Attia emphasizes the importance of focusing not just on quantity, but also on the quality of life. Happiness isn't just about adding years to your life; it's about adding life to your years. It's about experiencing joy, purpose, and fulfillment in every stage of your journey.

Felix Experience

Meet Felix the corporate cog. He doesn't miss a day at work, clocks in at 8, out at 8, rinse and repeat. Felix felt that he had a decent life, but was he happy? Felix later confessed to me that happiness was more like a distant memory to him and had no idea what happiness felt like anymore.

Then, his health was attacked. His cholesterol level was off the chart and he was going through immense stress even on the verge of a breakdown. The kind that gnawed at your insides, leaving you feeling hollow and exhausted.

His doctor suggested mindfulness along with other healthy living practices such as gratitude journaling, improving social connection, and even the art of kindness. Felix felt uneasy about the practice of mindfulness but he had no choice as his health was failing.

Felix signed up for a course, he was schooled on how to breathe and to focus on the present moment. With time, something shifted. The constant chatter in his head quieted, replaced by a sense of calm. His health improved drastically, he found a reason to wake up every morning and didn't feel it was a boring routine anymore but something he always looked forward to.

During one of his social outings, he met Matilda, six months later they were engaged and married today with two beautiful kids. Felix thanked the day he decided to be intentional about his life, today his life is like a fairy tale. It wasn't magic, though. It was hard work. Learning to control his thoughts, to let go of anxieties, and to appreciate the little things. But with each practice, the burden felt lighter.

Soon, the benefits spilled over. At work, he became more focused and less reactive. His relationship with colleagues at work improved, replaced by genuine connection, not just polite exchanges. And most importantly, he started to **enjoy** life again. The simple things began to matter, the sunrise, the smell of coffee, the laughter of friends – these simple joys have become precious moments today.

Today, Felix is not some Zen master. He still experiences bad days once in a while and even moments of doubt. But the difference is, he is now armed with the right coping mechanism.

With time, Felix began to see significant changes in his colleagues, friends, and even my family. People are catching on to the power of mindfulness, the magic of living in the present.

So, if you're feeling stuck, stressed, or just plain unhappy, take a chance. Give mindfulness a try. You might just discover, like Felix, that happiness isn't a destination, it's a journey. And it all starts with a single mindful breath.

CHAPTER 6: BEYOND HAPPINESS: BUILDING THE PILLARS OF WELL-BEING

Discovering the Relationship between Happiness, Nutrition, Exercise, and Sleep

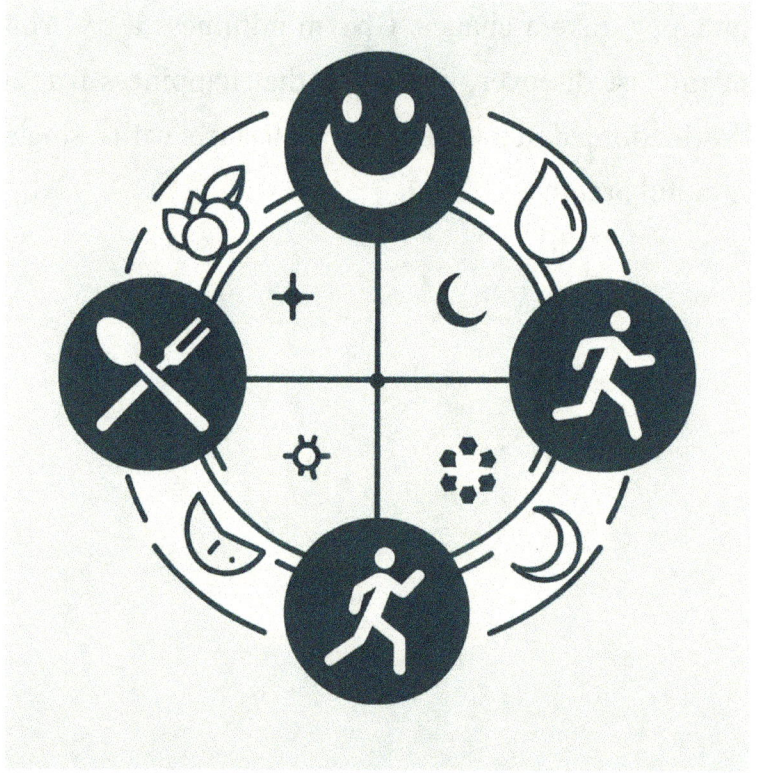

"Happiness and health are so closely related that it is difficult to tell which is the cause and which effect." - Alexis Carrel

While the pursuit of happiness remains a cornerstone of human existence, it's crucial to recognize that happiness alone is not enough for a fulfilling life. True well-being encompasses a broader spectrum, including robust physical and mental health, a sense of purpose, and strong social connections. This chapter delves into the interplay between happiness and three fundamental pillars of well-being: nutrition, exercise, and sleep.

Recent decades have witnessed a remarkable shift in life expectancy. What was once a rarity, living 100 years is becoming increasingly attainable thanks to advancements in various areas like healthcare, sanitation, and education. A child born today in developed countries has a 50% chance of reaching 104, compared to just 1% in 1914. This shift is not limited to a lucky few – it's becoming a global phenomenon.

While this is a cause for celebration, it also presents a crucial question: how can we ensure that these additional years are filled with health, well-being, and a sense of purpose?

While happiness is undoubtedly a crucial element of well-being, it's not the sole determinant of a long and fulfilling life. It's crucial to recognize that happiness is a dynamic state, influenced by various factors, including our physical and mental health. This chapter delves deeper, focusing on three key pillars that interact with happiness and form the foundation of holistic well-being: **nutrition, exercise, and sleep.**

Dr. Peter Attia challenges the conventional approach to health. His philosophy shifts the focus from mere lifespan extension to optimizing our overall well-being and maximizing the quality of our years. One of the core pillars of this approach is understanding the complex connection between happiness, nutrition, exercise, and sleep – factors intrinsically tied to both physical and emotional health.

Dr. Attia emphasizes a science-based approach, recognizing the powerful link between mental and physical health. Happiness, a complex blend of positive emotions and life satisfaction, isn't simply a fleeting feeling. Studies show it has tangible benefits for longevity. Happier individuals tend to have stronger immune systems, lower stress hormones, and reduced inflammation – all of which can combat age-related diseases. Moreover, happiness promotes healthy behaviors, motivating us to make better choices when it comes to what we eat and how we move our bodies.

Proper nutrition forms the foundation of a long and healthy life. Dr. Attia encourages a shift from a calorie-centric view to a nutrient-dense approach, emphasizing whole, unprocessed foods. He believes optimal nutrition helps regulate blood sugar, control inflammation, and nourish our bodies at the cellular level. Exercise, another vital pillar, isn't simply about weight loss. Dr. Attia stresses its role in boosting cardiovascular health, strengthening muscles and bones, and improving overall metabolic function. This contributes to longevity and minimizes the risk of chronic diseases.

Finally, Dr. Attia's focus on sleep underscores its essential role in overall well-being. Adequate sleep supports cognitive function, reduces stress, and allows for vital cellular repair and rejuvenation. Chronically disrupted sleep patterns are a significant risk factor for many age-related diseases and contribute to a diminished quality of life as we age.

Nutrition: Fueling Your Body and Mind

The human body is an intricate machine, and just like any machine, it requires the right fuel to function optimally. Unfortunately, the modern world is often filled with conflicting information and fad diets, making it easy to fall into the "cargo cult" trap of blindly imitating others without understanding the underlying principles. Here we are looking at science-backed approaches to nutrition and key principles for healthy eating. We'll move beyond restrictive diets and move into sustainable, personalized strategies that empower you to make informed choices about what you put on your plate.

Key Pillars to Enjoyable Nutrition

- **Whole Foods are the Foundation:** Base your meals around a colorful variety of minimally processed foods. This means lots of:
  - **Fruits and vegetables:** Aim for half your plate at each meal.
  - **Whole grains:** Think brown rice, oats, quinoa, whole-wheat bread.

- **Legumes:** Beans, lentils, chickpeas – versatile protein sources packed with fiber.
- **Nuts and seeds** for healthy fats and a satisfying crunch.

- **Focus on Quality Protein:** Include protein in most meals for fullness and muscle support. Opt for:

  - **Lean options:** Fish, poultry, tofu, low-fat dairy.
  - **Legumes (again!)** These do double-duty as both protein and excellent sources of fiber.

- **Healthy Fats, Not Fat-phobia:** Fats are essential! Prioritize:

  - Avocados, olive oil, and nuts/seeds for their anti-inflammatory properties.
  - Fatty fish like salmon, is packed with omega-3 fatty acids crucial for heart and brain health.

- **Listen to Your Body:** Practice mindful eating and tune into hunger and fullness cues. This fosters a positive body image and reduces overeating.

- **Hydration is Key:** Water plays a role in virtually every bodily function. Aim for 8 glasses a day as a starting point, and adjust up based on thirst and activity.

Going Beyond Restrictive Diets

- **Sustainability Matters:** Find a way of eating that feels enjoyable and fits your lifestyle. Rigid diets are hard to maintain and can lead to disordered eating down the line.

- **No Food is "Off-Limits":** Demonizing foods leads to cravings and guilt. Moderation, not deprivation, is key.

- **Progress, Not Perfection:** Slip-ups are normal! Focus on a pattern of healthy choices over time, not being perfect for every single meal.

- **Individualization is Key:** What works for one person may not work for the next. Consider allergies, intolerances, preferences, culture, and health conditions when forming your eating plan.

Tips to Make the Transition

- **Start small:** Choose one or two aspects to change at a time, don't overhaul everything at once.

- **Plan ahead:** Simple meal prep prevents unhealthy choices when you get hungry.

- **Crowd out, not restrict:** Focus on *adding* more whole foods rather than just *taking away* others.

- **Seek Support:** It could be a registered dietitian, an online community, or even a friend who shares your goals.

Important Considerations:

- **Talk to your doctor:** Especially if you have underlying health conditions, seeking professional guidance can be crucial.

- **Don't Confuse Wellness with Weight Loss:** Healthy eating offers numerous benefits beyond weight – improved energy, stable mood, and reduced risk of chronic diseases.

- **Be Kind to Yourself:** Body image and food issues are real. Consider seeking support if you struggle with a negative relationship with food.

Exercise: Building a Strong Foundation

Exercise isn't just about looking good; it's about building a strong foundation for both physical and mental health. It plays a critical role in reducing chronic disease risk, improving cognitive function, and enhancing mood. Let's explore the different forms of exercise, and the benefits of these exercises, helping you find a sustainable routine that fits your lifestyle and preferences. Remember, exercise isn't a punishment; it's an investment in your well-being, and finding activities you enjoy is key to long-term adherence.

Understanding Exercise: It's More Than Meets the Eye

Let's explore the different forms of exercise and the unique benefits each offers:

- **Endurance (Aerobic) Exercise:** Activities like brisk walking, running, swimming, dancing, or cycling get your heart pumping and your breathing elevated. These forms of exercise enhance cardiovascular health, improve stamina, manage blood pressure, and help maintain a healthy weight.

- **Strength Training:** Using resistance bands, weights, or your body weight, strength training builds muscle and bone density. This helps you maintain posture, reduce the risk of falls and injuries, boost metabolism, and improve your overall functional strength.

- **Balance Exercises:** Yoga, tai chi, and simple balancing exercises improve coordination and stability. Good balance prevents falls, a major risk factor for injuries as we age.

- **Flexibility Exercises:** Stretching, yoga, and other activities that focus on range of motion help keep your joints supple. Flexibility reduces stiffness, improves posture, and even eases everyday aches and pains.

The Benefits of Living a Long and Healthy Life

Regular exercise offers a vast range of benefits:

- **Physical Health:** Reduces risk of chronic diseases (heart disease, type 2 diabetes, certain cancers), improves sleep, reduces inflammation, enhances immunity, and helps with weight management.

- **Mental Health:** Boosts mood, lowers stress, sharpens memory, reduces anxiety and depression symptoms, and improves self-esteem.

- **Longevity:** It's directly linked to longevity, helping you live a longer and more independent life.

Find a Sustainable Routine and Make It Work for You

The key to success lies in finding activities you enjoy and that fit seamlessly into your lifestyle. Here's how:

- **Start Small:** Begin with short sessions, gradually increasing duration and intensity over time.

- **Be Kind to Yourself:** Don't push too hard too fast. Listen to your body and progress at a comfortable pace.

- **Mix It Up:** Explore different workouts to avoid boredom and prevent overuse injuries.

- **Find Your Tribe:** Exercise with a friend or join a class to stay motivated and accountable.

- **Make It Fun:** Choose activities you enjoy - dancing, gardening, hiking. You're more likely to stick with it long-term.

- **Lifestyle fit**: If gym visits aren't your thing, choose activities that fit your daily life – walking during lunch breaks, gardening, and bodyweight exercises at home.

- **Small steps = big results**: Even short bouts of activity throughout the day accumulate.

Important Reminders

- **Talk to Your Doctor:** Especially if you're new to exercise or have underlying health conditions.

- **Proper Form:** Focus on technique to prevent injury and maximize benefits. Look for videos or work with a trainer if needed.

Key Takeaway

Exercise is a powerful tool for a better, longer life. Find your unique rhythm with enjoyable activities – every movement counts, and it's never too late to start! Embrace the joy of exercise, and reap the rewards of long-term health and well-being.

Sleep: The Cornerstone of Restoration and Renewal

Sleep is not a luxury; it's a biological necessity. During sleep, our bodies repair and rejuvenate, solidifying memories and processing information. However, many of us struggle with getting enough quality sleep, leading to a cascade of negative consequences. Let's look at the science of sleep, debunk the common myths, and provide practical tips for achieving restful sleep and how it aids longevity. By understanding the importance of sleep hygiene and creating a sleep-conducive environment, you can unlock the restorative power of sleep and experience its transformative effects on your physical and mental well-being.

The Science of Sleep: Why It's Essential for Longevity

- **Cellular Repair and Regeneration:** During deep sleep, your body goes into overdrive repairing damaged cells, healing tissues, and fostering overall growth. This process is vital for maintaining a strong immune system and offsetting the wear and tear of daily life.

- **Hormonal Balance:** Sleep plays a crucial role in regulating essential hormones. Growth hormone (which aids in muscle and bone development) is primarily released during sleep, as is melatonin (which governs sleep-wake cycles). Imbalances can affect metabolism, weight, and general health.

- **Cognitive Function:** Sleep is when your brain consolidates memories, reinforces learning, and "cleans house" by removing waste products.

Lack of sleep leads to impaired attention, and problem-solving skills, and increased risk of cognitive decline later in life.

- **Disease Prevention:** Chronic sleep deprivation is linked to a higher risk of numerous health conditions including:
  - Heart disease
  - Stroke
  - Type 2 diabetes
  - Obesity
  - Some forms of cancer
  - Depression and other mood disorders

Debunking Sleep Myths

- **"I can catch up on sleep over the weekend":** Unfortunately, your body doesn't keep a sleep bank balance. While some recovery is possible, the effects of chronic sleep debt can't be entirely reversed with weekend sleep-ins.

- **"Alcohol helps me sleep":** Alcohol may make you fall asleep faster, but it disrupts your sleep cycle throughout the night, leading to less restful sleep and morning grogginess.

- **"Older adults need less sleep":** While sleep patterns may shift, the recommended 7-8 hours of quality sleep remains essential across all adult age groups.

- **"Napping is bad for nighttime sleep":** Short naps (20-30 minutes) for most people can improve alertness and focus. The key is to avoid long naps or naps late in the afternoon, as they might interfere with nighttime rest.

- **"Snoring is harmless":** While occasional snoring might be no big deal, loud or chronic snoring can be a major sign of obstructive sleep apnea, a serious condition where breathing repeatedly stops and starts during sleep. This disrupts oxygen flow and puts a strain on the body. Get it checked out!

- **"Napping makes nighttime sleep worse":** In fact, short naps (20-30 minutes) can improve alertness and performance without interfering with your nighttime rest. The key is to keep them brief and nap earlier in the day.

- **"If you can't fall asleep, staying in bed helps"**: Tossing and turning for too long can create anxiety around sleep. If you can't fall asleep within 20 minutes, get out of bed, do a relaxing activity in low light, and return to bed when you feel sleepy.

- **"Counting sheep helps you fall asleep"**: While trying to think yourself to sleep might seem productive, it can actually keep your mind racing. Try relaxing techniques like deep breathing or guided imagery instead.

- **"A nightcap helps you sleep better"**: As mentioned before, alcohol severely disrupts your sleep cycle, even if it makes you feel drowsy initially.

- **"You can train yourself to need less sleep"**: Some people are naturally shorter sleepers, but most adults truly do need around 7-8 hours. Chronic sleep deprivation has serious consequences, no matter how tough you think you are.

- **"Sleeping pills are the best solution for insomnia":** While they might be appropriate for short-term use in some cases, sleeping pills come with risks and side effects. Addressing underlying causes and improving sleep hygiene are better long-term strategies.

- **"You shouldn't exercise too close to bedtime":** For most people, moderate exercise is fine in the evening and can actually improve sleep quality. The exception would be high-intensity workouts right before bed.

- **"Waking up in the night means you have a sleep problem":** It's normal to wake briefly throughout the night as you transition between sleep cycles. As long as you can fall back asleep easily, it's usually nothing to worry about.

- **"The more sleep, the better":** Sleeping too much can disrupt your sleep-wake cycle and make you feel groggy. While some individuals might need slightly more than the average recommendation, excessive sleepiness could point to an underlying health issue.

Practical Tips for Restful Sleep & Enhanced Longevity

- **Consistency is King:** Stick to a regular sleep-wake schedule, even on weekends. This helps train your body's internal clock.

- **Set the Scene:** Your bedroom should be a sleep sanctuary:
    - **Cool:** Aim for a temperature around 60-67°F (15-19°C).
    - **Dark:** Use blackout curtains or an eye mask to block light.
    - **Quiet:** If possible, minimize environmental noise, or consider utilizing white noise or earplugs.

- **Wind-Down Routine:** Create a relaxing pre-sleep routine an hour before bed. This could include:
    - A warm bath or shower
    - Reading a calming book
    - Light stretching or meditation

- **Limit Screen Time:** The blue light from devices suppresses melatonin production. Aim to turn off screens an hour or two before bed.

- **Diet & Activity:**

    o Avoid heavy, spicy meals and large amounts of liquids before bedtime.

    o Limit caffeine, especially later in the day.

    o Regular exercise promotes better sleep, but avoid intense workouts close to bedtime.

The Importance of Sleep Hygiene

Sleep hygiene refers to the habits and behaviors that support healthy sleep. Good sleep hygiene is the foundation of achieving restorative sleep and promoting long-term health.

Lastly, if you struggle with chronic sleep difficulties, don't hesitate to consult a doctor or sleep specialist. They can help identify underlying conditions or recommend treatment options.

The path to greater happiness lies within our reach. By prioritizing nutritious whole foods, regular physical activity, and sufficient sleep, we take charge of our mental and physical health. These choices boost the production of feel-good brain chemicals, reduce stress, and enhance our emotional resilience. Remember, it's a journey, not a sprint. Embrace small, sustainable changes to cultivate a lifestyle that nourishes both body and mind.

CHAPTER 7: STRESS LESS, LIVE MORE
Practical Tools to Manage Stress and Cultivate Inner Peace

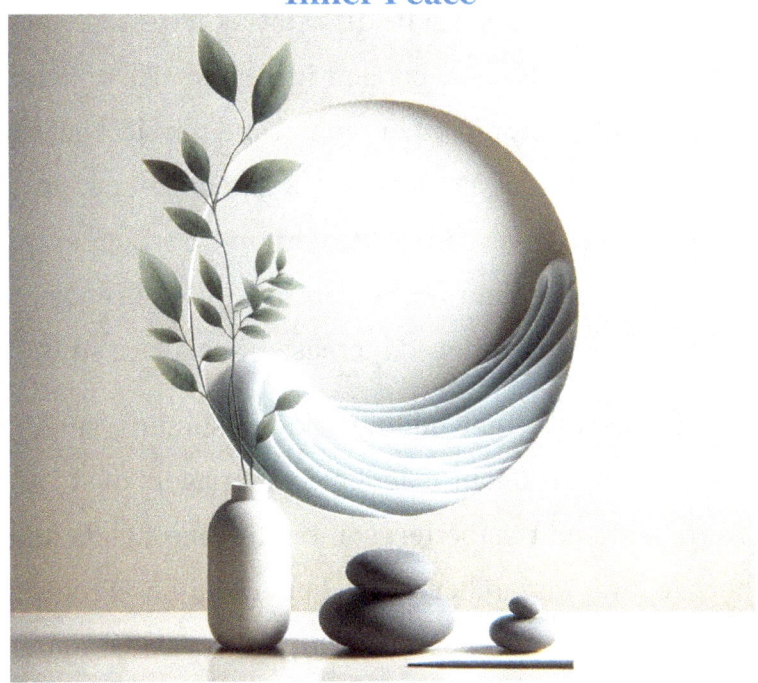

"Stress is not what happens to you, but how you react to it." - Hans Selye

"Stressed" spelled backward is "desserts." Coincidence? I don't think so. The opposite of vitality is stress. Across the globe, work-related stress levels are climbing, and with it comes a high number of health issues, from heart attacks to general disability. A recent study by the World Health Organization reported that the percentage of workers in the UK who say they are working 'very hard' or 'under a great deal of tension' had risen steadily since the 1980s. The results of this stress can be devastating. Stress at work is associated with a 20 percent increased risk of heart disease and a range of other mental and physical health issues. And this is not just a UK phenomenon. In a 2009 global survey of 1,000 corporations across 75 countries, more than 60 percent of workers reported that they had experienced increased workplace stress.

What is clear is that building and sustaining vitality assets is in part about managing the triggers of stress. To understand this better, some years ago Lynda and her fellow researcher Dr Hans-Joachim Wolfran studied over 200 people employed in complex, knowledge-based work. They found that being at work and being at home were not hermetically sealed existences. Rather, most people experience emotional spillover between the two places and the effect of this spillover could have a positive or negative impact on stress and therefore vitality.

You experience positive emotional spillover when you leave home in the morning feeling supported and relaxed and take these positive feelings into work; you leave work later in the day feeling productive, having learned new skills and built interesting networks and bringing these positive emotions and resources into the home. The emotional flow between work and home can also be negative. You leave home feeling tired and guilty, the kids are unhappy and you know that you are not giving your partner the support and encouragement they need. As you start working, these negative feelings of guilt and exhaustion immediately spill over and influence how you feel about the day ahead and the tasks you want to perform. This lack of emotional resources and vitality harms creativity and innovation, and in the long term leads to increased stress and the erosion of vitality.

Getting to experience the positive aspects of home (support and relaxation) rather than the negative (exhaustion and guilt), and the positive aspects of work (productivity, new skills, interesting networks) rather than the negative (frustration and boredom) depends on your choices and decisions. Fundamentally it comes down to the choices and decisions you make about the work you do, how you negotiate your role with your partner, and the way you allocate your time.

Understanding Stress

Stress is a natural physiological response to perceived threats or challenges. When we encounter stressful situations, our bodies release hormones like cortisol and adrenaline, preparing us for "fight or flight." This response is essential for survival in the short term, but chronic stress can have detrimental effects on our physical and mental health.

The Cost of Chronic Stress:

Chronic stress can manifest in various ways, impacting your:

- **Physical health:** Weakened immune system, increased risk of heart disease, high blood pressure, headaches, digestive issues, and sleep problems.

- **Mental health:** Anxiety, depression, fatigue, irritability, and difficulty concentrating.

- **Overall well-being:** Reduced quality of life, decreased productivity, and strained relationships.

Identifying Your Stressors

Before we can tame the stress monster, we need to understand its instruments. What are the specific situations, thoughts, or experiences that trigger your stress response? Are they deadlines, difficult conversations, financial worries, or something else entirely? Recognizing your individual stress triggers is the first step toward managing them effectively.

Here are some common stress triggers to consider:

- **Work:** Long hours, demanding tasks, difficult colleagues, lack of control, and job insecurity can all contribute to workplace stress.

- **Relationships:** Conflict, communication issues, and lack of support from loved ones can be significant stressors.

- **Finances:** Debt, job loss, or unexpected expenses can create significant financial strain and stress.

- **Health:** Chronic illness, injuries, or caring for a loved one with health issues can be physically and emotionally draining.

- **Major life changes:** Moving, divorce, death, or other major life changes can be stressful even if they are positive.

- **Negative thoughts:** Perfectionism, rumination, and catastrophizing can fuel stress and anxiety.

Once you have identified your personal stress triggers, you can begin to develop strategies for managing them.

Practical Tools for Managing Stress

Now that we know the instruments and the conductor, it's time to learn how to conduct the orchestra of stress. Here are some practical tools you can use to manage stress and cultivate inner peace:

- **Mindfulness and meditation:** These practices help you become more aware of your thoughts and feelings without judgment, allowing you to let go of negativity and focus on the present moment.

- **Relaxation techniques:** Deep breathing, progressive muscle relaxation, and guided imagery can help to calm your mind and body.

- **Exercise:** Regular physical activity is a powerful stress reliever and can also improve mood and sleep.

- **Healthy sleep habits:** Getting enough quality sleep is essential for both physical and mental health.

- **Time management:** Learn to prioritize tasks, set realistic goals, delegate work whenever possible, and learn to say no to requests that would overload you.

- **Positive self-talk:** Challenge negative thoughts and replace them with positive affirmations.

- **Social support:** Connect with friends, family, and loved ones who can offer support and encouragement.

- **Healthy eating:** Eating a nutritious diet can help to improve your mood and energy levels.

- **Humor:** Laughter is a great stress reliever, so find ways to incorporate humor into your life.

- **Seek professional help:** If you are struggling to manage stress on your own, don't hesitate to seek professional help from a therapist or counselor.

Cultivating Inner Peace

Managing stress is just one part of the equation. Cultivating inner peace is equally important for living a fulfilling and vibrant life. Here are some practices that can help you cultivate inner peace:

- **Manage Reactions**: Develop healthy coping mechanisms to manage stress instead of letting it take control. Learn techniques like deep breathing, progressive muscle relaxation, and positive self-talk.

- **Compassion:** Practice kindness and understanding towards yourself and others.

- **Living in the present moment:** Focus on what is happening right now, rather than dwelling on the past or worrying about the future.

- **Acknowledge Your Feelings**: Allow yourself to experience and process your emotions without judgment. Bottling emotions creates internal tension.

- **Identify Stressors**: Become aware of the events, situations, and thoughts that trigger stress responses in your life.

- **Forgive Yourself:** Practice self-forgiveness for past mistakes. Holding on to regret and guilt drains your energy.
- **Treat Yourself Kindly:** Prioritize activities that bring you joy and a sense of fulfillment. Engage in hobbies, spend time in nature, or connect with loved ones.
- **Shift Focus:** Regularly focus on the good things in your life, no matter how small. This trains your brain to notice the positive and combat negativity.
- **Gratitude Journal:** Keep a journal where you write down things you're grateful for. This cultivates a more appreciative outlook.
- **Exercise:** Regular physical activity releases endorphins, reduces stress, and improves overall health – all contributing to longer life.
- **Nutrition:** A balanced diet plays a crucial role in physical well-being and also influences mental and emotional health.
- **Sleep:** Adequate sleep is essential for both physical and mental restoration.

- **Acceptance:** Practice acceptance of what you can't control. Trying to manage every outcome in life creates anxiety and stress.
- **Focus on Your Actions:** Invest energy in what you can influence, such as your choices and reactions.
- **Seek Support:** Connect with friends, family, a therapist, or a spiritual community. Sharing burdens and having a support network is crucial.
- **Limit Unhealthy Distractions:** Minimize exposure to excessive news, negativity on social media, or other stressors that upset your inner peace.
- **Purpose:** Having a sense of purpose in life can provide direction and meaning.

Remember, there will be ups and downs along the way, but by incorporating these tools and practices into your life, you can learn to navigate them with more grace and resilience.

Jane's Experience

Call me the "Stress Queen! Okay, so maybe "queen" is a bit strong. But let's just say I'm well-acquainted with stress. It's like a clingy roommate who never leaves, always hovering, whispering worries in my ear. Deadlines loom, emails pile up, and the to-do list mocks me with its endless scribbles. My shoulders hunch, my jaw clenches, and before I know it, I'm in the clutches of full-blown stress mode.

Sound familiar? You're not alone. In this fast-paced world, stress seems to be a universal language. But here's the thing: we don't have to accept it as our default setting. Just like I learned to evict that overstaying roommate (okay, maybe not literally, but you get the idea!), we can learn to manage stress and cultivate inner peace.

I won't lie, it wasn't easy. I tried everything: gulping coffee, powering through late nights, even resorting to those sugary "stress relief" treats (which probably added more stress than they relieved!). But then I stumbled upon something different: practical tools and practices that helped me manage the stress monster.

Mindfulness became my mantra. Learning to be present in the moment, observing my thoughts and feelings without judgment, was a revelation. It was like stepping off the hamster wheel of worry and taking a deep breath. Suddenly, the world wasn't so overwhelming anymore.

But mindfulness wasn't enough on its own. I also needed to address the root causes of my stress. So, I started identifying my triggers – those pesky deadlines, the never-ending emails, the feeling of being constantly pulled in a million directions. Once I knew what was pushing my buttons, I could start to push back.

I learned to say "no" more often, delegate tasks, and prioritize ruthlessly. I carved out time for activities that brought me joy, like yoga and spending time with loved ones. Slowly but surely, the stress started to loosen its grip.

It wasn't an overnight transformation. There are still days when the worries creep in and I feel the familiar tension rising. But now, I have a toolkit of strategies to combat them. I can do some deep breathing, remind myself of what truly matters, and choose to focus on the present moment.

So, if you're feeling like the "Stress Queen" too, don't despair. There's hope! Remember, you're not alone in this. With the right tools and a little effort, we can all learn to manage stress and cultivate inner peace. And who knows, maybe someday we can all graduate from "Stress Queen" to "Inner Peace Empress." Now that's a title I could get behind!

CHAPTER 8: PENNYWISE, LIFEWISE
Making Wise Choices for Long-Term Happiness and Well-being

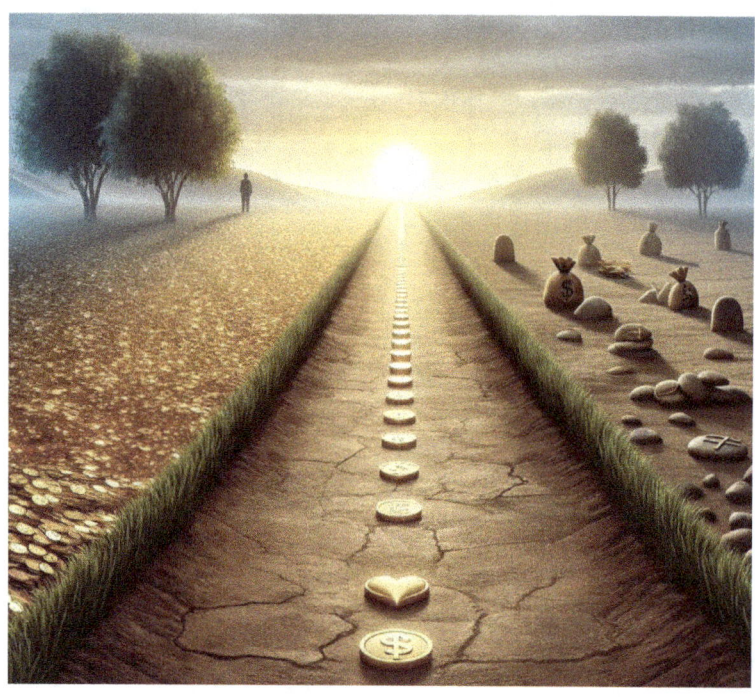

"True wealth is not measured in gold and silver, but in the richness of our relationships, the depth of our character, and the integrity of our lives." - Gautama Buddha

Many of us believe that the more we possess, the happier and more fulfilled we will be. However, an overabundance of research paints a different picture. A comprehensive study conducted by American Express among Baby Boomers revealed a fascinating truth: Americans prioritize experiences and relationships over material wealth in their definition of success. The survey highlights that:

- Americans define success by their actions and accomplishments, not their possessions. This is evident in the ranking of "having a lot of money" at a mere 20th place on the list of 22 factors contributing to a successful life.

- The vast majority (81%) believe knowing how to spend money wisely is a far greater indicator of success than simply having it in the first place.

- The vast majority (72%) prefer spending money on experiences over material things.

These findings are further supported by the fact that Americans now value a job they love, rewarding relationships, and contributing to their communities over accumulating wealth. When asked to rank the top contributors to a successful life, Americans prioritized:

1. **Being in good health (85%)**
2. **Finding time for the important things in life (83%)**

3. Having a good marriage/relationship (81%)
4. Knowing how to spend money wisely (81%)
5. Having a job you love (75%)
6. Making time to pursue passions and interests (69%)
7. Being physically fit (66%)
8. Always trying to learn and do new things (65%)
9. Embracing new experiences/changes (65%)

Interestingly, while a majority (57%) still aspire to become rich, it ranks #8 on America's bucket list, falling below learning how to be a better cook. This shift in values highlights a crucial point: true fulfillment comes not from material possessions, but from a life filled with meaningful experiences and connections, this can be one of the factors responsible for the decline in their mortality rate

(U.S. life expectancy from 1950 to 2024. United Nations projections are also included through the year 2100. The current life expectancy for the U.S. in 2024 is 79.25 years, a 0.18% increase from 2023. The life expectancy for the U.S. in 2023 was 79.11 years, a 0.08% increase from 2022. The life expectancy for the U.S. in 2022 was 79.05 years, a 0.08% increase from 2021. The life expectancy for the U.S. in 2021 was 78.99 years, a 0.08% increase from 2020)

The data above shows a gradual increase in life expectancy in the United States from 2021 to 2024. Each year, there's been a small but consistent increment:

- In 2021, the life expectancy was 78.99 years.
- In 2022, it increased slightly to 79.05 years.
- In 2023, it rose to 79.11 years.
- By 2024, it reached 79.25 years.

This pattern suggests an ongoing improvement in life expectancy in the U.S., with each year experiencing modest growth compared to the previous one. The percentage increase each year is small, indicating a steady, albeit slow, rise in the average number of years a person is expected to live.

Imagine a life where you're not just surviving, but thriving. A life filled with purpose, joy, and deep connections, even in the later chapters. This chapter isn't about chasing millions or living a life of excess. It's about making **pennywise choices** that lead to **life-wise outcomes**. It's about understanding that true wealth extends far beyond the material and into the realm of well-being, fulfillment, and meaningful connections.

The Myth of More

The American Dream often paints a picture of happiness tied to material possessions and financial abundance. However, research consistently shows that more money doesn't necessarily translate to more happiness. The pursuit of wealth can often lead to stress, anxiety, and even strained relationships.

The story of the broker who never had a client say "enough" perfectly illustrates this point. We're constantly bombarded with messages telling us we need more, but the truth is that true fulfillment comes from living a life aligned with our values and purpose, not chasing an ever-receding finish line.

Shifting Our Focus

So, where do we start? The first step is to shift our focus from acquiring more to appreciating what we already have. This doesn't mean ignoring financial planning or responsibility, but rather approaching it with a mindful and intentional perspective.

The American Express survey highlights this shift perfectly. Americans ranked having a job they love, rewarding relationships, and contributing to their communities as more important for a successful life than having a lot of money. They also expressed a preference for spending on experiences over material things.

Living with Less, Living More

The story of downsizing the family home is a powerful example of how simplifying can lead to greater freedom and fulfillment. Letting go of material possessions can create space for new experiences, deeper connections, and a lighter, more intentional way of life.

Two Paths to Financial Independence

The story of Rowland, the son who embraced frugality and built a fulfilling life with limited needs, demonstrates another path to financial independence. While not everyone will choose his exact lifestyle, the key takeaway is that happiness and freedom are not solely defined by the amount of money we have.

Planning for the Future, Not Just Reacting

The difference between a fulfilling second life and one filled with financial strain often lies in **planning**. Instead of waiting until retirement to figure things out, take the time to establish a clear vision for your future, including your financial needs. Consider your longevity goals and create a realistic plan to achieve them.

Financial Planning: Turning Dreams into Reality

The story of the family dream, where inheritance went to charity rather than individual children, showcases a different approach to wealth distribution. This approach fostered self-reliance, encouraged giving back, and ultimately strengthened family bonds.

There's no one-size-fits-all approach to financial planning. The key is to develop a plan based on your unique circumstances, values, and goals. Talk to trusted advisors, gather information, and make informed decisions that align with your vision for the future.

Ten Guiding Financial Principles

1. **Create a written plan**: Don't rely on others to do it for you. Seek professional input, but ultimately own your plan.

2. **Seek diverse perspectives**: Talk to people you admire and learn from their experiences.

3. **Focus on your children's needs**: What will truly help them thrive and become independent?

4. **Don't overemphasize wealth preservation**: Focus on values and contributions, not just numbers.

5. **Beware of tax-focused strategies**: Prioritize long-term goals over short-term gains.

6. **Be Thorough**: Invest time and effort in creating a comprehensive, written plan that reflects your goals. Seek guidance from professionals to refine, legalize, and personalize it.

7. **Seek Inspiration**: Engage in conversations with individuals you admire and learn from their experiences. However, remember to filter their advice through the lens of your unique needs and aspirations.

8. **Prioritize Needs**: Base your plan on a clear understanding of your children's individual needs and what truly motivates them to become independent and responsible individuals.

9. **Rethink Priorities:** Don't be fixated on amassing wealth solely for the purpose of leaving it to your children. Focus on fostering their self-reliance and sense of purpose.

10. **Seek Balanced Advice**: While tax benefits are important considerations, avoid falling prey to excessive focus on tax avoidance strategies. Prioritize creating a plan that aligns with your

Longevity Goals And A Realistic Plan To Achieve Them

Instead of aiming for the broadest idea of "living longer", let's refine it into maximizing your *healthspan*. This means focusing on the years you live in good health, with energy, mobility, and mental sharpness.

Sample Goal: "I want to maintain my ability to hike independently, travel with ease, and engage fully in social activities for at least 15 more years."

Realistic Plan

Here's a breakdown of key areas and how to make your plan realistic:

1. Baseline Assessment

- **Full Medical Checkup:** Talk to your doctor about your current health status, genetic risks, and any conditions to manage proactively.

- **Fitness Test:** Get a sense of your current strength, cardio fitness, and flexibility. A trainer or physical therapist can help with this.

2. **Pillar #1: Nutrition**

- **No Fad Diets:** Focus on balanced whole foods, plenty of vegetables, fruits, and lean proteins. Consult a registered dietician for a personalized plan if needed.

- **Hydration:** Dehydration impacts energy and cognition. Aim for the recommended water intake for your needs.

- **Reduce Highly Processed Foods:** These offer little nutritional value and can worsen health conditions over time.

3. **Pillar #2: Exercise**

- **Mix it Up:** Include cardio (walking, swimming, cycling), strength training, and flexibility exercises.

- **Listen to Your Body:** Start at a comfortable intensity and gradually increase. Prioritize consistency over extreme workouts.

- **Find What You Enjoy:** This makes it far more likely you'll stick with it. Dance, group classes, outdoor adventures... find your fun ones!

4. **Pillar #3: Mental Wellbeing**

- **Stress Management:** Explore mindfulness practices, meditation, time in nature, and whatever works for you to reduce chronic stress.

- **Mental Stimulation:** Learn a new skill, do puzzles, read challenging books, and engage in social activities. Keep your brain active!

- **Purpose & Connection:** Strong social ties and a sense of purpose have enormous benefits for longevity.

5. **Pillar #4: Rest & Recovery**

- **Quality Sleep:** 7-8 hours is a must for most adults. Establish solid sleep hygiene.

- **Manage Medical Conditions:** Work closely with your doctor to treat any sleep apnea, restless leg syndrome, or other disruptors.

- **Listen to Your Body:** Schedule rest days from exercise, and allow sufficient recovery time.

Making it Realistic

- **Small Changes:** Start with 2-3 new habits at a time, don't overwhelm yourself. Focus on consistency rather than perfection.

- **Find Support:** Consider a walking buddy, a fitness class, or online groups for encouragement.

- **Track Progress:** This doesn't mean obsessing over numbers! Celebrate improved energy, being able to complete a harder hike, or remembering things more easily.

- **Regular Review:** Check in with yourself and your doctor annually to reassess and make adjustments.

Important Notes:

- Longevity is influenced by genetics, but lifestyle choices play a major role.
- This is a sample plan. Your specific needs may require adjusting it with professional help.
- Embrace the journey and the positive impact you're making on your health, not just the distant goal!

Answering the Right Questions

Before making financial decisions, ask yourself *"who, what, when, where, and why"* questions. Identify your beneficiaries, objectives, timelines, and motivations. Only then can you determine the "how" with the help of professionals.

Don't tie inheritances to specific conditions as that can have unintended consequences and hinder personal growth.

In conclusion, Financial planning is not just about numbers; it's about crafting a life filled with meaning, purpose, and well-being. By making pennywise choices, prioritizing experiences over possessions, and focusing on what truly matters, we can create a fulfilling and enriching future, not just for ourselves, but for generations to come.

Dave's Experience

I used to be a "buy now, pay later" kind of guy. A gadget freak who chased every new experience, always striving to keep up with the Joneses. But the relentless pursuit of stuff left me feeling empty and, ironically, broke. That's when I stumbled upon the concept of "pennywise" living – making smart choices with my money instead of letting it control me.

It wasn't easy at first. I had to break ingrained habits, confront my FOMO (fear of missing out), and redefine what "success" meant for me. It wasn't about keeping up with the latest trends or accumulating the most stuff, but about building a life filled with experiences and connections that truly mattered.

One of the first things I did was downsize. My elaborate apartment felt like a burden, sucking up a significant chunk of my income. Moving to a smaller, more manageable space liberated both my finances and my mind. Suddenly, I had more time and energy to explore things I genuinely enjoyed, like hiking and volunteering at a local animal shelter.

The joy of giving back replaced the fleeting satisfaction of buying material possessions. Witnessing the impact of my contributions brought a deeper sense of fulfillment than any new gadget ever could.

This shift wasn't about depriving myself; it was about making conscious choices. Instead of blindly following every marketing message, I learned to ask myself: "Do I truly need this? Will it bring lasting joy, or is it just a fleeting high?" This simple question became a powerful filter, helping me avoid unnecessary purchases and redirect my resources toward more meaningful pursuits.

One of the biggest lessons I learned was the importance of planning. I started crafting a financial roadmap, setting realistic goals, and seeking guidance from a trusted financial advisor. This empowered me to take control of my future instead of being a passive participant in the whims of the economy.

Today, I'm still figuring things out, but I'm no longer chasing an illusion. I've built a life that aligns with my values, one that prioritizes experiences, purpose, and connection over fleeting material pleasures. And the best part? This path to fulfillment is open to everyone, regardless of income level. It's about making conscious choices, prioritizing what truly matters, and living a life that's rich in meaning, not just possessions.

PART 3: LIVING A LIFE OF JOY: PUTTING IT ALL TOGETHER

CHAPTER 9: EMBRACING THE ZEN WITHIN
Integrating Mindfulness and Acceptance into Daily Life

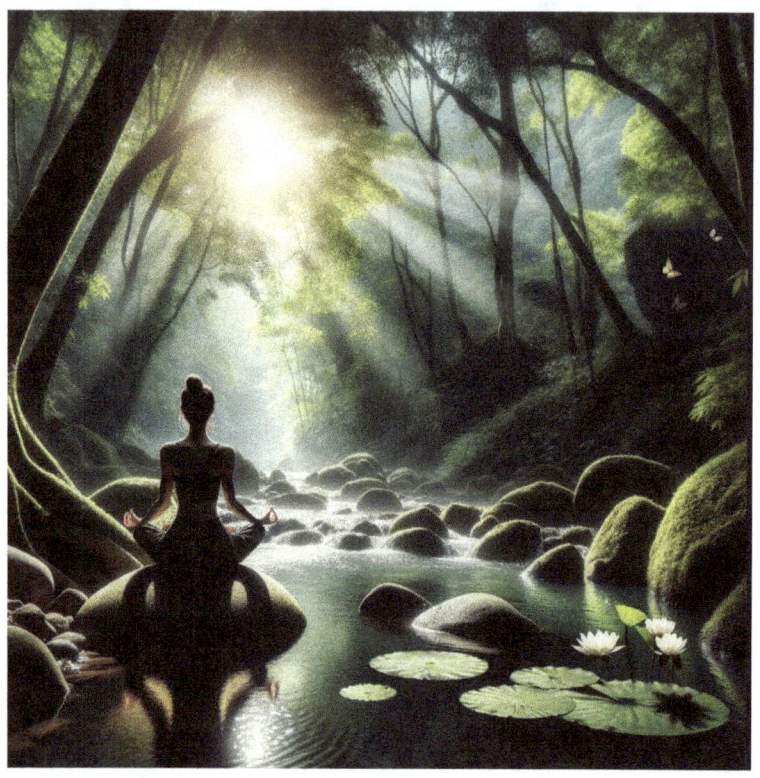

"One who looks around him is intelligent, one who looks within him is wise."– Matshona Dhliwayo

In the previous chapters, we explored various pillars of living a long and fulfilling life, emphasizing healthy habits, a strong social circle, and a sense of purpose. However, a crucial element often overlooked is the

inner world – our thoughts and how they impact our overall well-being. This chapter delves into the practice of **mindfulness and acceptance**, drawing inspiration from Zen principles, to help us navigate the inner landscape and cultivate greater joy in daily life.

Living in the "Now": The Power of Mindfulness

The human mind is a curious thing. It can be a powerful tool for creativity, problem-solving, and planning for the future. However, it can also become a source of suffering if we constantly dwell on past regrets, anxieties about the future, or negative self-talk. This constant mental chatter, often disconnected from the present moment, can significantly impact our happiness and well-being.

Mindfulness is the practice of bringing our attention to the present moment without judgment. It involves observing our thoughts, feelings, and bodily sensations with an open and curious mind, rather than getting caught up in them. Think of it like stepping back from the constant stream of thoughts and simply observing its flow without feeling the need to control or judge.

The Benefits of Mindfulness

Research suggests that mindfulness practice offers a lot of benefits:

- **Reduced stress and anxiety:** By anchoring ourselves in the present moment, we can distance ourselves from worry and rumination about the past and the future, leading to a calmer and more peaceful state of mind.

- **Improved focus and concentration:** Mindfulness teaches us to be aware of distractions and gently redirect our attention back to the present moment, leading to better focus and concentration in daily tasks.

- **Enhanced emotional regulation:** By observing our emotions without judgment, we can learn to manage them more effectively, preventing them from controlling our actions and reactions.

- **Increased self-awareness:** Through mindfulness, we gain a deeper understanding of our thoughts, feelings, and motivations, allowing us to make more conscious choices aligned with our values.

Integrating Mindfulness into Your Daily Life

Mindfulness isn't about achieving a state of perfect stillness or emptying your mind. It's a practice that takes time and effort to cultivate. Here are some simple ways to incorporate mindfulness into your daily routine:

- **Mindful breathing:** Take a few minutes each day to simply focus on your breath. Feel the rise and fall of your chest as you inhale and exhale. When your mind wanders, gently bring your attention back to your breath without judgment.

- **Mindful eating:** Instead of eating mindlessly while watching TV or working, take the time to savor your food. Pay attention to the colors, textures, and tastes. Eat slowly and deliberately, enjoying each bite.

- **Mindful walking:** As you walk, pay attention to the sensations in your body - the feeling of your feet hitting the ground, the movement of your arms, and the breeze on your skin. Be aware of your surroundings – the sights, sounds, and smells.

- **Mindful moments throughout the day:** Throughout your day, take small moments to be present. As you wash your hands, feel the warmth of the water and the scent of the soap. As you answer the phone, take a deep breath and listen attentively to the person on the other end.

Acceptance: Embracing the Present Moment

Mindfulness is closely linked to the concept of **acceptance**. Acceptance doesn't mean passively accepting all negative situations or giving up on improvement. Instead, it involves acknowledging our current reality – our thoughts, feelings, and circumstances – without judgment or resistance.

Why is acceptance important? Often, we struggle because we fight against reality. We want things to be different than they are. This resistance can create additional suffering and prevent us from moving forward. By accepting the present moment, we can find a sense of peace and clarity, even amidst challenges.

Integrating Acceptance into Your Daily Life

Here are some ways to cultivate acceptance in your daily life:

- **Observe your thoughts and feelings without judgment:** Don't label your thoughts and feelings as good or bad. Simply acknowledge them and let them go.

- **Accept that things are temporary:** Everything in life is constantly changing. Accepting this impermanence can help us let go of attachment to specific outcomes and embrace the flow of life.

- **Focus on what you can control:** While we can't control external circumstances, we can control our reactions and actions. Focus your energy on what you can influence, and let go of trying to control what you can't.

Combining Mindfulness and Acceptance: A Path to Joy

By integrating both mindfulness and acceptance into our daily lives, we can cultivate a sense of **inner peace, clarity, and joy**. This combined practice allows us to navigate the ups and downs of life with greater resilience and equanimity.

How Mindfulness and Acceptance Work Together

Imagine yourself standing on the shore, watching the waves roll in and out. The **mindful** perspective would involve observing the waves without judgment, noticing their size, shape, and sound. The **acceptance** perspective would involve acknowledging the ocean's current state, and understanding that the waves are constantly changing and beyond your control.

By combining these two perspectives, you can observe the waves without getting swept away by them. Similarly, in life's journey, you can observe your thoughts and emotions with awareness while accepting the present moment without resistance. This allows you to respond to situations calmly and with greater wisdom, rather than being controlled by them.

Benefits of Combining Mindfulness and Acceptance:

- **Reduced reactivity:** By observing your thoughts and feelings with awareness, you can choose your response rather than automatically reacting in a way that may later cause regret.

- **Increased self-compassion:** Accepting your thoughts and emotions without judgment fosters self-compassion, allowing you to treat yourself with kindness and understanding even during difficult times.

- **Enhanced emotional well-being:** By acknowledging and accepting your emotions, you can move through them without getting stuck or overwhelmed by them.

- **Greater resilience:** When faced with challenges, acceptance helps you let go of resistance and adapt to changing circumstances with greater ease.

Putting It All Together

Here are some strategies to combine mindfulness and acceptance in your daily life:

- **Mindful self-compassion:** During moments of self-criticism, practice mindful observation of your thoughts and feelings. Acknowledge them with kindness and understanding, reminding yourself that everyone experiences challenges and imperfections.

- **Mindful acceptance of difficult emotions:** When experiencing negative emotions like anger or sadness, observe them without judgment. Recognize that these emotions are natural and temporary, and they don't define you.

- **Mindful acceptance of challenges:** When facing difficult situations, acknowledge the challenge without fueling resistance or negativity. Practice mindful observation of your thoughts and emotions, and focus on taking one step at a time through the situation.

Consistent practice is key to developing the skills of mindfulness and acceptance. As you integrate these practices into your daily life, you'll cultivate greater inner peace, joy, and resilience, allowing you to navigate through life's challenges with greater wisdom and grace.

EXERCISE 3: Embrace Your Inner Zen: A Fun and Practical Exercise

Let's explore the power of these practices in cultivating inner peace and navigating life's ups and downs. Now, it's your turn to put these concepts into action.

1. **The Present Moment Quiz:**

Test your mindfulness skills with this quick quiz! Answer the following questions based on your current experience, right now, at this moment:

- What are 3 things you can see around you? (It could be the color of the walls, a picture on the desk, or even your own hand!)

  _____
  _____
  _____

- What are 2 sounds you can hear? (Is it traffic outside, the hum of a computer, or maybe your own breathing?)

  _____
  _____
  _____
  _____

- What 1 physical sensation can you feel? (Is it the feeling of your clothes against your skin, the chair beneath you, or the coolness of the air?)

_____

_____

2. My Mindful Moment:

Take a few minutes to practice mindfulness in your own way. Here are some ideas:

- **Mindful breathing:** Close your eyes and focus on your breath. Feel your chest rise and fall with each inhale and exhale. If your mind wanders, gently bring your attention back to your breath. (You can set a timer for 2-3 minutes)

- **Mindful walking:** Take a walk around your house or outside, paying attention to the sensations in your body and your surroundings. Notice the way your feet feel against the ground, the sights you see, and the sounds you hear.

- **Mindful eating:** If it's mealtime, choose a healthy snack and savor it mindfully. Pay attention to the colors, textures, and tastes of your food. Eat slowly and deliberately, enjoying each bite.

3. **Acceptance Challenge:**

Think about a situation in your life that is causing you stress or frustration. Now, try to approach it with acceptance:

- Acknowledge your thoughts and feelings about the situation without judgment.

- Remind yourself that things are constantly changing, and this situation is temporary.

- Focus on what you can control in the situation, and let go of trying to control what you can't.

4. **Share your experiences!**

- Did the mindfulness exercise help you become more present in the moment?

_____
_____
_____
_____
_____

- What challenges did you face during the acceptance challenge?

  _____
  _____
  _____
  _____

- How can you integrate mindfulness and acceptance into your daily routine?

  _____
  _____
  _____
  _____

CHAPTER 10: ONE STEP AT A TIME

Building a Sustainable Path Towards a Happy and Fulfilling Life

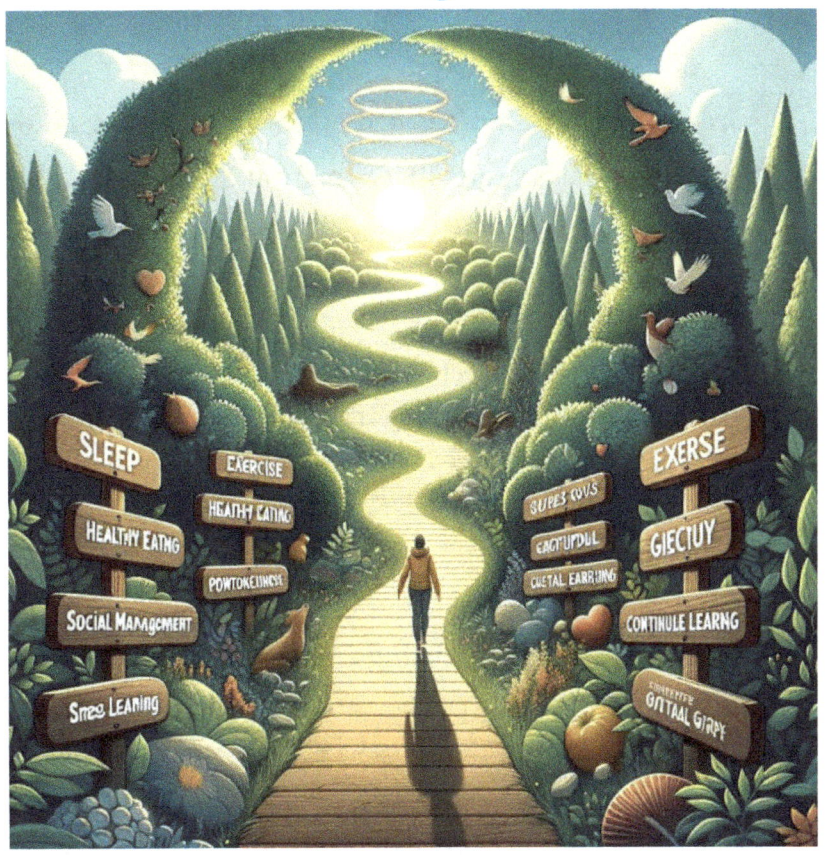

"The journey of a thousand miles begins with a single step." - Lao Tzu

Life is a marathon, not a sprint. While we all dream of achieving grand goals and living a life filled with joy and fulfillment, the process can often feel overwhelming. We get caught up in the desire for instant gratification, comparing ourselves to others, and chasing fleeting happiness. However, true and lasting happiness and fulfillment come from building a sustainable path, one step at a time.

Drawing inspiration from the teachings of Dr. Peter Attia and other experts in longevity and well-being, this chapter will guide you through practical steps you can take to lay the foundation for a happy and fulfilling life, starting today.

The Power of Small, Sustainable Habits

Our brains are wired for habit formation. The things we do repeatedly, whether good or bad, become ingrained in our neural pathways, making them easier to do over time. This is why focusing on **small, sustainable habits** is crucial for lasting change.

Research supports this approach. Studies have shown that individuals are more likely to stick with long-term behavior changes when they start small and gradually increase the difficulty as they build confidence and momentum. For example, aiming to add just 10 minutes of daily walking instead of aiming for an hour-long workout right off the bat is far more likely to become a sustainable habit.

Here's why small habits are so powerful

- **Feasible and Achievable:** Small habits are easier to integrate into your daily routine and require less willpower to maintain, making them more sustainable in the long run.

- **Cumulative Effect:** Over time, even small changes can lead to significant improvements in your overall health and well-being.

- **Momentum Builder:** Completing small habits can boost your confidence and motivation, encouraging you to take on bigger challenges and build upon existing positive changes.

Applying the "One Step at a Time" Approach to Different Aspects of Your Life:

Now that you have a foundation, it's time to start building! Here are some practical steps you can take to cultivate a happy and fulfilling life, drawing inspiration from Dr. Attia's work:

1. Prioritize Sleep: Adequate sleep is fundamental for both physical and mental health. Aim for 7-8 hours of quality sleep each night.

2. Cultivate Healthy Eating Habits: Focus on whole, unprocessed foods, fruits, vegetables, and lean protein sources. Remember, small improvements can make a big difference. Maybe swap out sugary drinks for water or add a daily serving of vegetables to your meals.

3. Move Your Body Regularly: Aim for at least 150 minutes of moderate-intensity exercise or 75 minutes of vigorous-intensity exercise per week. Find activities you enjoy, whether it's brisk walking, dancing, or joining a team sport.

4. Build Strong Social Connections: Humans are social creatures, and strong relationships contribute significantly to happiness and well-being. Nurture your existing connections and actively seek opportunities to build new friendships.

5. Manage Stress: Chronic stress can negatively impact your physical and mental health. Explore various stress-management techniques like mindfulness meditation, yoga, or spending time in nature.

6. Practice Gratitude: Taking time to appreciate the good things in life, both big and small, can shift your perspective towards positivity and well-being. Consider keeping a gratitude journal or taking a few minutes each day to reflect on what you're grateful for.

7. Embrace Continuous Learning: Never stop learning and growing. Engage in activities that stimulate your mind, whether it's reading a book on a topic you find interesting, taking a class, or learning a new skill.

8. Give Back to Others: Helping others can significantly contribute to your own sense of purpose and fulfillment. Volunteering your time, donating to a cause you care about, or simply being kind to others can make a difference.

There will be bumps along the road, and that's okay. The key is to be patient, celebrate your progress, and keep taking one step at a time.

The Power of Consistency

The magic lies in consistency. Even small, seemingly insignificant steps, when taken consistently over time, can lead to significant and sustainable improvements in your overall well-being and happiness.

Focus on Progress, Not Perfection

Strive for progress, not perfection. Don't get discouraged by setbacks or occasional slip-ups. Everyone makes mistakes, and what matters most is that you learn from them and keep moving forward.

Celebrate Your Wins

Taking even small steps toward your goals is worthy of celebration. Acknowledge your progress, no matter how small, and reward yourself for staying on track. This positive reinforcement will help you stay motivated and committed to your journey.

Tips to help you stay on track

1. **Find an Accountability Partner:** Sharing your goals and progress with a trusted friend, family member, or coach can provide valuable support and keep you motivated.

2. **Focus on the Process, Not Just the Outcome:** Enjoy the journey of making positive changes and learning new things, rather than solely focusing on the end result. This can help you stay engaged and motivated in the long run.

3. **Seek Inspiration:** Read stories of individuals who have overcome challenges and achieved their goals. Surround yourself with positive and inspiring people who can motivate you on your journey.

4. **Embrace Setbacks as Learning Opportunities:** View setbacks as opportunities to learn and grow. Analyze what led to the setback and adjust your approach accordingly. Remember, progress is not always linear, and setbacks are a natural part of the learning process.

5. **Practice Self-Compassion:** Be kind and understanding towards yourself. Acknowledge your efforts and celebrate your progress, even when things don't go according to plan. Treat yourself with the same compassion and understanding you would offer to a friend in a similar situation.

6. **Focus on the Positives:** When faced with challenges, actively seek out the positive aspects of your situation. Reframing negative thoughts into a more positive light can significantly impact your overall outlook and motivation.

7. **Remember Your "Why":** Regularly revisit your core values and goals. Remind yourself why you embarked on this journey and what truly matters to you. Renewing your commitment to your values and aspirations can provide a source of strength and motivation when faced with challenges.

Building a happy and fulfilling life is not about reaching a specific destination; it's about embracing the journey itself. By taking one step at a time, prioritizing your well-being, and nurturing your values, you can cultivate a life filled with meaning, purpose, and lasting happiness. Remember, the choices you make every day, however small they may seem, contribute to the overall direction of your life. So, choose wisely, celebrate your progress, and enjoy the beautiful journey of living a long and fulfilling life.

Janes Experience

For a long time, my life revolved around a little pill called Tramadol. It started innocently enough. A bike accident left me with a nagging knee injury, and my doctor prescribed Tramadol to help me manage the pain. At first, it seemed like a miracle cure. Not only did it ease my physical discomfort, but it also had this strange side effect of numbing my worries and anxieties.

Before I knew it, I wasn't just taking Tramadol for my knee. I was taking it to go to work, to socialize, to even run basic errands. The pills became a crutch, a way to cope with the everyday stresses of life. I told myself it was fine because it was a prescription medication. Doctors knew what they were doing, right?

The turning point came when I realized I couldn't function without Tramadol. If I ran out or forgot a dose, panic would set in. The dull ache of withdrawal would creep over me, a mix of physical pain and a crushing sense of unease that made it impossible to focus on anything else. That's when I knew I was dependent, that the medication was controlling me, not the other way around.

The idea of quitting was terrifying. I'd heard the horror stories about opioid withdrawal. But staying on that path was even more frightening. I knew I could lose my job, my relationships, and ultimately, myself.

I didn't go cold turkey. I'd tried that before and the withdrawal was unbearable. Instead, I decided to take it one step at a time. I talked to my doctor and we devised a plan to slowly taper off my dosage. It was a long, difficult process. There were days when the cravings were overwhelming, days when my body ached and my mind raced. The first few days were rough. My body protested, and withdrawal symptoms crept in – restlessness, nausea, and that gnawing anxiety returned with a vengeance. But I stayed the course, taking those steps – one shaky one after the other.

But I held on. I reached out to support groups, found a therapist, and leaned on a few trusted loved ones who knew my secret. Slowly but surely, the fog of Tramadol began to lift. I rediscovered forgotten joys— reading a book without getting distracted, and laughing with friends without feeling the need to numb myself.

It wasn't a perfect, straight line of progress. There were setbacks and slip-ups. But through it all, I kept reminding myself why I was doing this. I envisioned the life I wanted, a life free from the shackles of addiction.

Today, I'm proud to say I'm off Tramadol. The journey was one of the hardest things I've ever done, but also one of the most rewarding. I've learned so much about myself, about resilience, and about the power of taking things one step at a time. There are still challenges, of course, but I face them head-on without the crutch of a pill. And looking forward, I know I have so much ahead of me – possibilities I couldn't see while Tramadol clouded my judgment.

CHAPTER 11: THE JOURNEY CONTINUES

Spreading Lifetime Happiness, Embracing Continuous Growth, And Building Connections For A More Meaningful Life

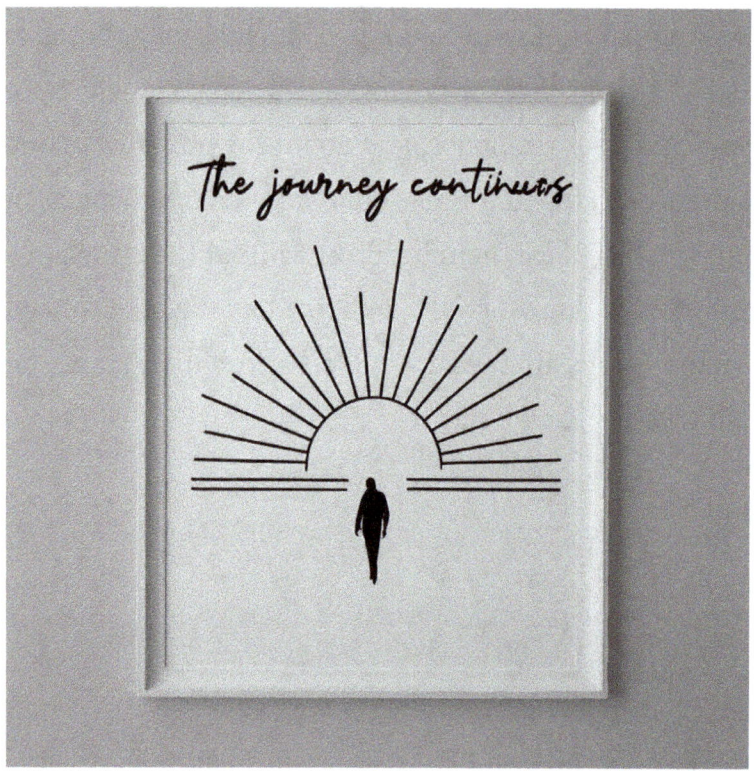

"The purpose of life is not to be happy. It is to be useful, to be honorable, to be compassionate, to have it make some difference that you have lived and lived well." – Duane Mayes

Life is a journey filled with experiences, challenges, and opportunities for growth. While we strive for happiness and longevity, it's equally important to consider how we can make this journey meaningful and impactful not just for ourselves, but for others as well. This chapter, inspired by Dr. Peter Attia's teachings on health and well-being, explores how we can cultivate lifetime happiness, embrace continuous growth, and build strong connections for a more fulfilling and purposeful life.

Spreading Lifetime Happiness: The Ripple Effect of Positivity

Dr. Attia emphasizes the importance of optimizing health as a foundation for a long and fulfilling life. However, true happiness extends beyond physical well-being. It involves cultivating positive emotions like joy, gratitude, and compassion. These positive emotions have a ripple effect, influencing not only ourselves but also those around us.

Research suggests that acts of kindness can:

- **Boost your own happiness:** Helping others releases feel-good hormones like dopamine and oxytocin, leading to increased feelings of joy and connection.

- **Strengthen relationships:** Acts of kindness foster trust, compassion, and a sense of belonging, strengthening the bonds you have with others.

- **Create a more positive environment:** When kindness becomes contagious, it can create a ripple effect, fostering a more positive and supportive environment for everyone.

Examples of Spreading Happiness

- Offer to help someone in need, whether it's holding a door open, assisting with a grocery bag, or offering to listen to a friend who's going through a tough time.

- Practice random acts of kindness, like leaving a positive note for a stranger, donating to a cause you care about, or volunteering your time.

- Express gratitude to those who have made a positive impact on your life, letting them know how much you appreciate them.

Embracing Continuous Growth: A Lifelong Journey of Learning

Life is filled with opportunities to learn and grow. By embracing continuous learning, you can expand your knowledge, develop new skills, and challenge yourself in new ways. This not only keeps your mind sharp and engaged but also fosters a sense of personal accomplishment and boosts your overall well-being.

Dr. Attia encourages a proactive approach to learning, seeking information and experiences that can help you optimize your health, relationships, and overall well-being. This can include:

- **Reading books and articles on various topics that interest you.**
- **Taking online courses or workshops to develop new skills and knowledge.**
- **Engaging in stimulating conversations with people from diverse backgrounds and perspectives.**
- **Stepping outside your comfort zone and trying new things, even if they seem challenging at first.**

Remember, learning is a lifelong journey. Don't be afraid to make mistakes and view setbacks as opportunities for growth. Embrace the excitement of discovery and the joy of expanding your horizons.

Building Connections: The Power of Strong Relationships

Humans are social creatures, and strong, meaningful connections are essential for a fulfilling life. These connections provide us with a sense of belonging, support, and love, contributing significantly to our overall well-being.

Here's how to nurture strong connections:

- **Invest time and effort in your existing relationships:** Make time for regular communication with family and friends, even if it's just a quick phone call or a short message.

- **Be present and engaged in your interactions:** Put away distractions and actively listen to others, showing genuine interest in their lives and experiences.

- **Practice empathy and compassion:** Strive to understand the perspectives and feelings of others, offering support and encouragement when needed.

- **Expand your social network:** Seek opportunities to meet new people, join clubs or groups that share your interests, and step outside your comfort zone to build diverse connections.

Building strong connections requires effort and intentionality. By investing time and energy in nurturing your relationships, you can create a supportive network that adds significant meaning and richness to your life.

Life's journey is not about reaching some ultimate destination but rather about the experiences and connections we create along the way. By spreading happiness, embracing continuous learning, and building strong connections, you can contribute to a more meaningful and fulfilling life for yourself and those around you. Remember, the journey continues, and every step you take toward becoming a better, happier version of yourself is a step toward a life filled with purpose and joy.

CONCLUSION

Happiness isn't just about feeling good in the moment. It's a powerful force that fuels our health and extends our time on Earth. Throughout this book, we've explored how happiness works, and how to build it into our lives.

Before you go, remember these key lessons:

- **Happiness is yours to define.** Don't let anyone tell you what should make you happy.
- **Self-compassion is key.** Quieting your inner critic helps you grow and make better choices.
- **Happiness is just one part of the puzzle.** Nourish your body with healthy food, move regularly, and get enough sleep.
- **Stress is your enemy.** Find healthy ways to manage it, and your overall well-being will improve.
- **Mindfulness matters.** Being present in each moment brings joy.
- **The journey never ends.** Embrace a lifetime of learning, growing, and connecting with others.

True longevity is about more than just living a long life. It's about filling those years with joy, purpose, and genuine connection. This book has given you the tools; now it's your turn to create a long and truly happy life.

Bonus: Q&A: Unlock Your Awesome Life

1. **Q: What's the main idea of "The Art of Longevity"?** A: It's a guide for living a longer, healthier, and happier life.

2. **Q: Who should read this book?** A: Anyone interested in improving their health, extending their lifespan, and finding more joy in life.

3. **Q: What makes this book different from others on longevity?** A: It focuses on practical steps, not just scientific theory.

4. **Q: What's the most important factor for longevity?** A: Healthy habits are key - diet, exercise, sleep, and stress management.

5. **Q: Does diet matter that much?** A: Yes! What you eat has a huge impact on your health and lifespan.

6. **Q: What's the best exercise for longevity?** A: A mix of cardio (like walking) and strength training (like lifting weights).

7. **Q: How much sleep do I need?** A: Most adults need 7-8 hours of good quality sleep each night.

8. **Q: How can I handle stress better?** A: Mindfulness, meditation, and finding healthy outlets are important.

9. **Q: Does staying positive help me live longer?** A: Yes! Optimism and a sense of purpose are linked to a longer lifespan.

10. **Q: Should I retire early for a longer life?** A: Not necessarily. Staying engaged and active can be beneficial.

11. **Q: How do strong relationships help me?** A: Social support reduces stress and improves your overall health.

12. **Q: Do supplements help with longevity?** A: Some are helpful, but always talk to your doctor first.

13. **Q: What about anti-aging medicine?** A: Some new treatments show promise, but more research is needed.

14. **Q: Should I get regular health checkups?** A: Absolutely! Early detection of problems is key to a longer life.

15. **Q: Can I reverse aging?** A: Not completely, but you can slow it down.

16. **Q: How long can humans live?** A: The maximum lifespan isn't certain, but healthy habits increase yours.

17. **Q: Can I start making changes later in life?** A: Yes, it's never too late to improve your health!

18. **Q: Is this book just for old people?** A: Nope! Good habits benefit you at any age.

19. **Q: What if I'm afraid of getting old?** A: The book helps you reframe aging as a positive process of growth and learning.

20. **Q: How do I find meaning in my later years?** A: Focus on giving back, pursuing passions, and staying connected to loved ones.

21. **Q: Is it normal to worry about death as I get older?** A: Yes, the book offers ways to approach thoughts about mortality with peace.

22. **Q: What about the physical challenges of aging?** A: The book provides strategies for

maintaining mobility, independence, and a positive outlook.

23. **Q: How can I cope with losing loved ones as I age?** A: It covers healthy grieving, finding support, and cherishing memories.

24. **Q: Do genetics determine how long I'll live?** A: Genetics play a role, but lifestyle choices have an even greater influence.

25. **Q: Can I change my habits even if I've been unhealthy?** A: Absolutely! Even small changes make a big difference over time.

26. **Q: I feel overwhelmed, where do I start?** A: The book offers simple steps and helps you choose one area to focus on at a time.

27. **Q: Are there 'shortcuts' to longevity?** A: No, but there are science-backed habits that make the process easier.

28. **Q: Will following this book guarantee I live to 100?** A: No, but it greatly increases your chances of a long, healthy, and happy life.

29. **Q: Does longevity mean sacrificing all joy?** A: Not at all! The book is about maximizing enjoyment and living fully.

30. **Q: Do I need to be rich to follow this advice?** A: No, many longevity-boosting habits are free or affordable.

31. **Q: Can I still be happy if I'm dealing with a chronic illness?** A: Yes! The book includes ways to adapt, find joy, and thrive even with health challenges.

32. **Q: What if I don't have much time left?** A: The book helps you focus on what matters most and make the most of your time.

33. **Q: Is this book about avoiding death?** A: No, it's about embracing life fully, including its natural end.

34. **Q: What specific areas of science are advancing longevity research?** A: Genetics, cellular biology, regenerative medicine, and anti-aging technologies.

35. **Q: Are there promising medications that might extend lifespan?** A: Some emerging

drugs target aging processes, but more research is needed.

36. **Q: What role does technology play in longevity research?** A: AI, big data analysis, and wearable tech are revolutionizing how we track health and potentially slow aging.

37. **Q: Are there ethical concerns with longevity research?** A: Yes, including issues of access, overpopulation, and potential unintended consequences.

38. **Q: How might increased longevity affect society?** A: It could change retirement systems, healthcare, and family structures.

39. **Q: Could extending lifespan worsen inequality?** A: Yes, if access to longevity treatments is limited to the wealthy.

40. **Q: What are the environmental implications of longer lifespans?** A: Potential strain on resources needs to be balanced with innovation.

41. **Q: How can governments prepare for a population with more older adults?** A:

Proactive policies around healthcare, pensions, and age-friendly communities.

42. **Q: How can I learn more about my own longevity potential?** A: There are genetic testing options and tools for assessing your biological age.

43. **Q: What practices from long-lived cultures ("Blue Zones") can I incorporate?** A: Prioritize plant-based diets, strong community, and daily movement.

44. **Q: Can cryonics (freezing the body) really extend life?** A: It's highly speculative and relies on future, unproven technology.

45. **Q: Is radical life extension desirable for everyone?**
A: It sparks personal and philosophical debates about the meaning of life.

46. **Q: How does mental health affect longevity?** A: Depression, anxiety, and chronic stress significantly shorten lifespan.

47. **Q: Does spirituality play a role in a long life?** A: For many people, faith provides purpose, community, and stress reduction.

48. **Q: What is the role of creativity in longevity?** A: Creative pursuits keep the mind engaged and may protect against cognitive decline.

49. **Q: How can I prepare for the 'fourth age' (80+)?** A: Focus on financial planning, staying socially connected, and potential long-term care.

50. **Q: What are some reliable sources for staying updated on the latest longevity research?** A: Reputable journals (like Nature, Cell), science-focused websites (e.g., ScienceDaily), and dedicated longevity organizations offer trustworthy information.

www.ingramcontent.com/pod-product-compliance
Lightning Source LLC
Chambersburg PA
CBHW050248010526
44107CB00003B/234